Comments on **Multiple sclerosis at your fingertips**
from readers

'My overall impression is of excellence and comprehensiveness. The thoroughness of the approach is much needed, as MS is so complex and individual.'

Jan Hatch,
Director of MS Services, **MS Society**

'I found it easy to read and understand. My wife Pam, who is 47, could easily relate to much of the contents.'

Allan Quartley, Somerset

'Having explored numerous treatments, both conventional and so-called "alternative", I find your book provides the information necessary to make an educated decision on how to follow up any treatments or therapies. In brief, it is delightful to find a book that does not go into so much medical detail as to make it incomprehensible to the lay person, yet still covers the various options that an MS sufferer has available in the management of the illness. What I found most useful is that it is a book that you can give to your relatives and friends in order to ease their comprehension of the illness.'

Edith J. Pasternak-Albert

Reviews of **Multiple sclerosis at your fingertips**

'Having been sent a copy for review, I "road tested" it, looking at the sections covering employment, mobility, speech problems and alternative therapies. I thought the book was indeed valuable, giving as it did very sensible, detailed information. The chapter headings were clear. There was an index and a glossary of terms associated with the condition – no need to be flummoxed when your neurologist gets technical about CAT scans or dyplopia.'

MS Scotland
(newsletter of the
Multiple Sclerosis Society, Scotland

'This book will help those who want to understand the complexity and individuality of multiple sclerosis. It allows readers to explore elements of the disease with appropriate advice and lifestyle adjustments. This book encourages health professionals to take a positive approach to managing patients with MS. The chapters on "You and your family" and "Other relationships" cover very important aspects of MS which are sometimes neglected. Close family requires as much education and reassurance as the patient. "Problems with urination and bowels" is delicately explained with plenty of practical tips on bladder management.'

Nursing Times

Multiple sclerosis at your fingertips

THE MEDICALLY ACCURATE MANUAL WHICH TELLS YOU ABOUT MS AND HOW TO DEAL WITH IT

Ian Robinson MA
Director of the Brunel MS Research Unit, Department of Human Sciences, Brunel University, West London

Dr Stuart Neilson BSc, PhD
Lecturer in the Department of Epidemiology and Public Health at University College Cork, Eire [and former Director of Medical Information Systems at the Centre for the Study of Health, Sickness and Disablement (CSHSD), Brunel University]

Dr Frank Clifford Rose FRCP
Consultant Neurologist, London Neurological Centre, Harley Street, London

CLASS PUBLISHING • LONDON

2000

Printing history
First published 2000
Reprinted 2000

The author and publishers welcome feedback from the users of this book.
Please contact the publishers.
Class Publishing, Barb House, Barb Mews, London W6 7PA, UK
Telephone: (020) 7371 2119
Fax: (020) 7371 2878
email: post@class.co.uk
web site: http://www.class.co.uk

A CIP catalogue record for this book is available from the British Library

ISBN 1 872362 94 X

Designed by Wendy Bann

Cartoons by Jane Taylor

Illustrations by David Woodroffe

Edited by Michèle Clarke

Indexed by Val Elliston

Production by Landmark Production Consultants Ltd, Princes Risborough

Typesetting by Martin Bristow

Printed and bound in Finland by WS Bookwell, Juva

Contents

Note to reader

As you read this book, you will find that some words are in *italic*. These are highlighted to inform you that explanations can be found in the Glossary at the back. If you are looking for particular topics, use either the detailed list of Contents on pp. v–vii or the Index which starts on p. 235.

Foreword

by Jan Hatch

Director of MS Services, Multiple Sclerosis Society
of Great Britain and Northern Ireland

Every day seven people are diagnosed with multiple sclerosis. Some of them will be relieved because, after years of living with invisible and mysterious symptoms, fear and confusion, they will finally have a label for their condition. For others the diagnosis will be a devastating shock, presenting difficulties and problems far beyond the effects of the disease itself.

MS is an unpredictable disease, affecting everyone who has it differently. No one can say what the future impact of the disease on any one person will be. This uncertainty about the future and the unpredictability of the present is the most disabling aspect of MS, and that is why accurate information is so important to people with MS. Reliable and comprehensive answers to the wide range of questions that people with MS have will enable them to make informed decisions about their present and future.

This book will be an invaluable resource to many people who are living with this chronic, fluctuating disease. It will answer their questions, sensibly and comprehensively, and will enable them to take as much control as they can of their own lives. The information contained in this book is the most important tool a person can have in managing the effects of multiple sclerosis. It will give them the power to make choices for themselves.

Jan Hatch

1
Multiple sclerosis explained

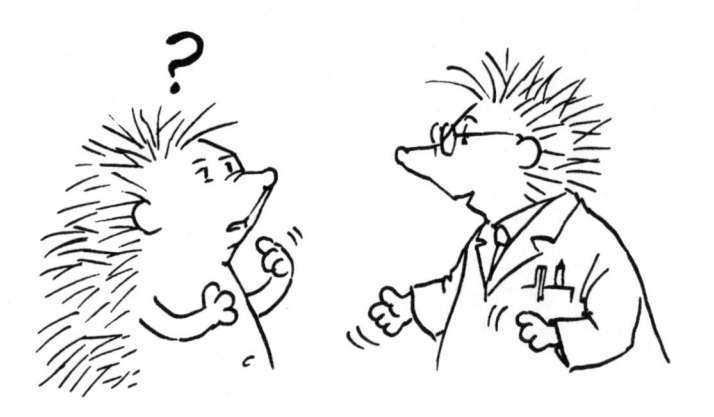

This chapter explains the current scientific and medical under-standing of the disease. We begin with a description of what multiple sclerosis (MS) is; we then provide some information about the *epidemiology* of the disease (the geographic and demographic distribution of people who currently have MS, and how these patterns are changing); finally we discuss different types of MS.

What is MS?

MS is a disease of the central nervous system (CNS); it damages the protective coating around the nerves (*neurons*) (Figure 1.1) which transmit messages to all parts of your body, especially to do with the control of muscular and sensory activity. It is thought to be an *autoimmune disease*: this is where your body's own immune system appears to attack itself. As the damage to the protective coating around the nerves – called *myelin* – increases, it leads to a process known as *demyelination* (Figure 1.2), where the coating is gradually destroyed. These nerves then become less and less efficient at transmitting messages. The messages, as it were, 'leak' from the nerves where demyelination has occurred, rather like the loss of an electric current through a cable that is not insulated. As the messages 'leak', they become weaker and more erratic, thus leading to greater and greater difficulty in controlling muscles or certain sensory activities in various parts of your body.

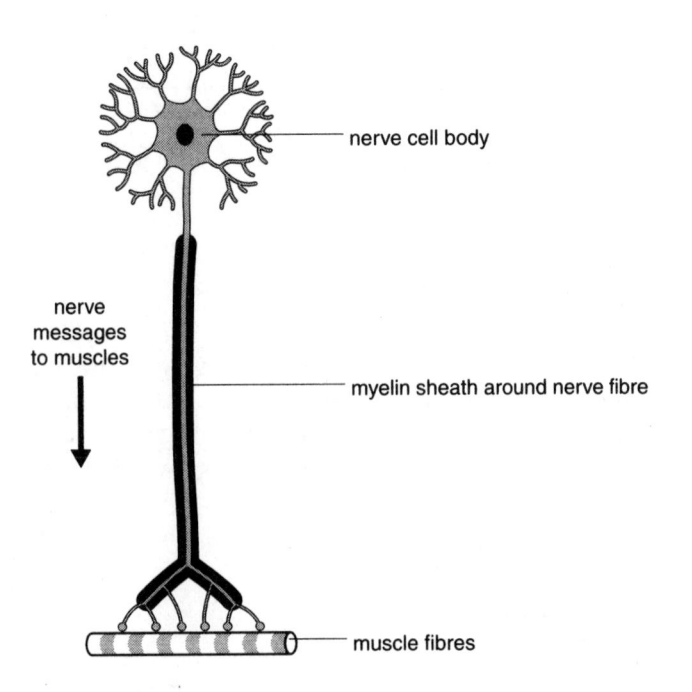

Figure 1.1 Normal neuron.

However, which nerves are demyelinated, in which order, and at what rate, varies very widely between individuals, so the corresponding loss of muscular and sensory control also varies widely. Moreover, even when damage does occur to the myelin, it is gradually repaired (i.e. remyelination occurs) through internal body repair mechanisms; also, what might be described as 'inflammation' at the site of the damage often becomes less over time. However, in MS the rate of repair is slower than the rate at which the myelin is damaged; so the damage tends to accumulate more and more throughout the central nervous system. This damage results in plaques or lesions, which take the form of patchy scarring (*multiple scleroses*) where the demyelination has occurred. Thus the name 'multiple sclerosis' has evolved.

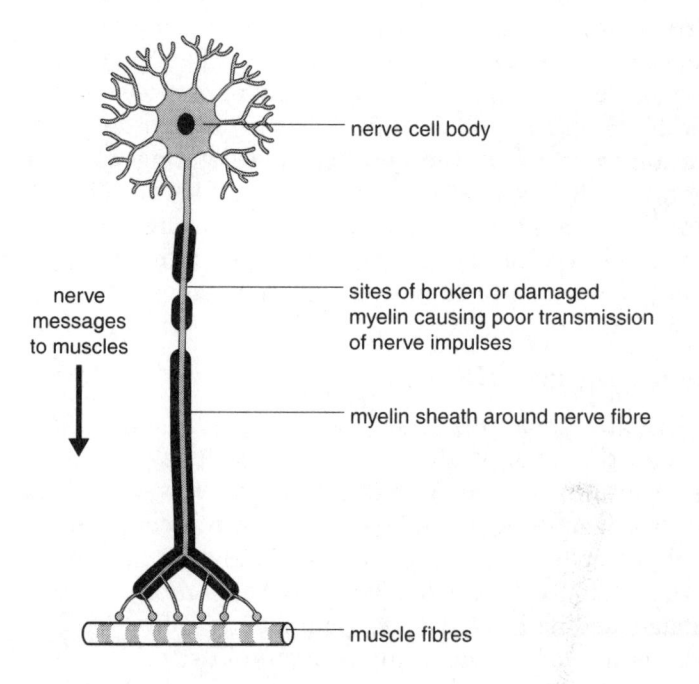

Figure 1.2 Demyelination of neuron.

How many people and who can get MS?

How many people have MS?

It is difficult to give an exact number, because we cannot be sure that everyone who has MS has been diagnosed with the disease. However, based on a range of epidemiological studies (studies which investigate the distribution and patterns of disease in the community), it seems most likely that there are around 85 000 people who currently have MS in the UK. This means that roughly one in every 1000 people has the disease. This is called the *prevalence* of MS (the number of people who have been diagnosed and are currently alive with the disease). As to the *incidence* (the number of new cases that are added to this pre-existing prevalence 'pool' of people with MS every year), approximately 2500 people are added, or seven people every day. It must be stressed, however, that these figures are essentially informed 'guesstimates' based on extrapolations from smaller-scale local and regional studies. There are no detailed studies covering everyone in the country, investigating whether or not they have MS. The cost of doing so would be prohibitive. So the overall figures of both incidence and prevalence may change over time if new studies suggest that the patterns of MS are different from those previously thought to exist.

Who usually gets MS?

Statistically speaking people are usually diagnosed with MS between the ages of 20 and 50, and so it is considered to be primarily a disease of young adults. However, MS can occur outside this age range, but it is less likely to occur – although it is not impossible – the younger you are under 20, and the older you are over 50. Most studies have shown that more women tend to be diagnosed with the disease than men (a ratio of 1.7 women to 1 man is the most commonly reported in studies). The disease also seems to be more common in white people than in black Africans (or African-Caribbeans) or in most people of Asian origin. Geographically it appears that people who are living in the more temperate, cooler latitudes are more liable to develop MS, and it is very uncommon in tropical or semitropical areas of the world.

Why is MS so common in some parts of the world compared to others, the Faroe Islands for example?

One of the interesting and important features of MS, which has triggered much research, is its uneven distribution throughout the world. MS appears to be more frequent amongst white populations, amongst people of North European descent, and amongst people with particular blood groups. MS is more frequent in Europe and North America than most of Africa and Asia. The Faroe Islands, which are small islands situated in the North Atlantic and governed by Denmark, appear to have had the highest prevalence of MS in the world in relation to their population in the post-World War II period, and have been the subject of intense research. The prevalence of MS in the Faroes, however, as well as the incidence, has been declining since the 1960s. In this situation research has not unnaturally focused on something which happened during, or shortly after the War, that might have triggered the rapid increase in MS. Much interest has been targeted on a period of occupation by UK military forces; it has been vigorously argued by some that they brought with them a viral trigger that raised local rates of MS. The lengthy and still unresolved debate over this issue is one of the most celebrated in the history of MS research, and will probably only be resolved with other conclusive evidence, yet to be gained, about the general cause(s) of MS (see Chapter 3).

On a more general point, the prevalence of MS is greater the further away from the equator you go (towards the poles). This *latitude effect* may be related to some underlying genetic similarities; to lifestyle factors and longevity in the more affluent populations in the Northern and Antipodean nations; to environmental factors, or to other disease characteristics of these populations, such as the later age at which children are generally first exposed to many viral diseases in these countries; this is thought by some to give less 'immunity' to the subsequent development of diseases such as MS. However, these ideas are now being reconsidered in the light of very recent evidence that the latitude differences are declining. They may also possibly have arisen in the first place from the better health surveillance of developed nations, and were just what is known as an *artefact effect*, i.e. the latitude differences were never real differences, but just came about through the inaccurate ways in which we measured them. Now there is some evidence that those latitude differences may actually be reversed in some individual countries, including the UK, where recent research suggests that the prevalence of MS is greater in the South than in the North.

Is MS becoming more common?

In many recent studies of the extent of MS, numbers of recorded cases of the disease appear to be higher than in previous surveys made in exactly the same, or a similar geographical area, so it seems that MS is becoming more *prevalent*, i.e. there are now more people with MS. Furthermore, the numbers of people with MS in the UK have more than doubled in the past three decades. However, we must be clear about this change; it does not mean that more people are 'catching' MS – it is not infectious – or that some other cause (inherited or environmental) has led to many more people having the condition. The increase is attributable to several other factors.

- Improvements in health services, and particularly in the availability of referrals to neurologists, have led to an increase in the number of people, who already had MS in the community, now being formally and correctly diagnosed with it – this is what is described as *improved case ascertainment*. In addition, it is possible that there may have been an increase in the speed of diagnosis, i.e. people who already have MS are being diagnosed at younger ages than previously.

- There is a very general effect of *population ageing*, from better overall health and longer life expectancies, which has led to an expansion in the proportion of the population aged 25–65 years when MS is most frequent.

• People with MS now have a far better life expectancy themselves than in the past; for example, they now live approximately 11 years longer than people with MS did three decades ago. A greater medical awareness of the disease process, particularly of some of the serious symptoms that occur when MS is more severe, and the availability of better treatments, especially antibiotics, have made this improvement possible.

Are women at greater risk of catching MS?

First, just to be clear again, MS cannot be 'caught'. It is not an infectious disease. However, as we have noted, more women are diagnosed overall, with a ratio of about 1.7 women with MS for every man with the disease. Women also tend to be diagnosed at a younger age, and thus there is an even greater difference in the sex ratio below the age of 30 years, i.e. there are far more women than men with MS under 30. In relation to older ages, men are more likely than women to experience their first symptoms after the age of 40, and also to have the *chronic progressive* type of the disease (see later in this chapter). It is quite likely that some of these differences may be related to underlying biological and hormonal differences between the sexes, although the nature of the links is not yet precisely clear.

There is no evidence of any excess risk, compared to the general risk of having MS, amongst men or women unrelated to you 'by blood', such as marital partners, adopted children and so forth. However, women who are related to someone with MS by close blood ties, i.e. mothers, daughters and sisters, do have an increased risk of developing MS. Closely related men also show this increased risk, but it is slightly higher in women because of the higher proportion of women who tend to have MS. (For further information about the genetic aspects of MS, see the section on *Genetics* in Chapter 3.)

Can children get MS?

The overwhelming majority of cases of MS occur after the age of 15. Exceptionally, people are referred with MS-like symptoms at younger ages, but are usually diagnosed after the age of 15. If you, or someone you know, has MS-like symptoms at 15 or younger, then the chances are that it is not MS. However, the symptoms should be followed up, as many other conditions can produce symptoms like MS. These are mostly everyday and temporary, but a few can be very serious, and even fewer fatal if untreated. All these other conditions are more common than MS in young teenagers.

There are other conditions that young children may have, in which the process of demyelination is in common with MS, but they are not related to MS, are exceptionally rare, and are usually inherited – but through a different genetic profile than that which is associated with MS (see Chapter 3).

Types of MS

How many different types of MS are there, and what distinguishes each of them?

To be perfectly frank, it could be said that there are almost as many different forms of MS as there are people with the disease. Each person with MS has a slightly different clinical (and symptom) profile; the precise course that any one person's MS will take is not as predictable with the kind of detail that many people with the condition – as well as their doctors – may wish for. In this context, scientists and doctors are always trying to refine their classification of types of MS, as they get to know more and more about the condition and its symptoms. You may therefore come across several slightly different ways of describing types of MS.

Nevertheless, it can be useful to identify several general 'types' of MS that most doctors would recognize and that have broad characteristics in common, but in many cases – given the variability of the disease – it is not possible to classify easily the particular 'type' of MS you may have in its very early stages.

- Most cases of MS are generally described as *relapsing-remitting*, especially in younger people. Symptoms worsen during an 'attack' or 'relapse', may be at their worst for several days or a little longer, and then gradually improve in the following weeks. Some attacks or relapses may lead to a permanent decrease in the abilities affected, whilst in others, especially in the early stages of the disease, the *remission* or recovery may be almost complete. 'Dampening down' a relapse, as well as recovery after one, can be helped by the use of *immunosuppressive drugs*, although it is still unclear whether short-term success in their use has a significant effect on the long-term course of MS over 10 years or more. Something like two-thirds of people with an initial relapsing-remitting history of MS find that their symptoms have become progressive within 15 years of diagnosis, as the length of time during relapses increases and the number and duration of remissions decrease. The disease is then said to take a *secondary progressive form*.

- *Chronic progressive* (or *primary progressive*) MS describes another pattern of the disease in which symptoms gradually worsen after the first 'episode' or 'attack', with a continuing increase in disability, often in bodily movement (described as *motor symptoms*) of one kind or another, or in sensory performance (especially eyesight). With this type of MS, which is relatively rare, serious disability can occur over a few months, but in most cases MS will progress over many years or decades with a very much slower increase in disability. Nevertheless, in this type of MS, 'remissions' do not occur, and it is possible that in due course serious speech difficulties, and other problems may arise. Chronic progressive MS affects about one-fifth of all people with the disease, and is more common amongst those who experience their first symptoms after the age of 40 years. About one-third of the people with the initial gradual but unrelenting chronic progressive course of MS find that the symptoms begin to worsen significantly and rapidly progress within the first five years.

- *Benign MS* is a term sometimes used to describe a course of MS in which symptoms are relatively minor, or progression is so slow that it is almost clinically imperceptible, or there are very few attacks or relapses over long periods of time – usually 15 years following diagnosis. Although mild attacks or relapses may occur infrequently in benign MS, recovery, from the point of view of symptoms, seems usually to be almost complete and with no worsening of disability. However, the term should be used very warily, for it is essentially a statement about how the MS has progressed so far in an individual; it may not be a useful indicator of how the MS will progress in the future, particularly given the notorious unpredictability of the disease. Indeed, some recent research has concluded that, over even longer periods of time (25 years following diagnosis and beyond), most of those people who were originally described as having benign MS have developed significant disability.

- Finally, just in case you hear this point from other sources (but don't worry about it unduly), there is what some think to be a very, very rare variant of MS, but which others think might be a separate disease, that can lead to death in a few months. The causes of death are the same as those that may be precipitated by other forms of MS. This rare form is sometimes, although completely misleadingly, described as malignant MS, for it has nothing at all to do with cancer with which the term 'malignant' is usually associated.

2
Symptoms of MS

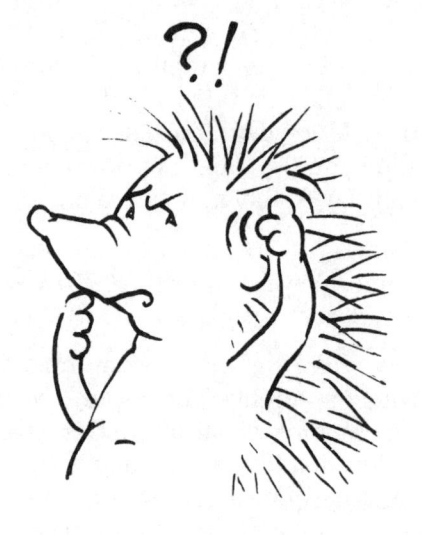

There are many symptoms associated with MS that occur to a greater or lesser degree. Some are more debilitating than others; some cause more inconvenience. They can, for example, include problems with:

- urinary and bowel function (Chapter 7)
- pain and changes in sensation and dizziness (Chapter 8)
- tiredness (Chapter 9)
- depression and cognitive or memory impairment (Chapter 9)
- mobility (Chapter 10)
- speech and eating difficulties; problems with eyesight and hearing (Chapter 11).

Symptom management in MS is often a complicated process. The symptoms may occasionally be wide ranging and so variable that a variety of strategies are often required: from lifestyle changes; drug therapies; psychological or counselling support; particular physio, speech and occupational therapies; use of equipment; environmental modifications; to surgery in some cases. Many symptoms may involve more than one of these strategies, depending on their seriousness. The main concern for all those involved in managing your symptoms, including you and your family, is to find an appropriate balance between all the strategies, especially when several symptoms occur simultaneously.

This introductory chapter talks about MS symptoms before and after diagnosis. More detailed discussions are given in the chapters listed above on the most important symptoms that may affect you and their day-to-day management.

What are the usual symptoms of MS? How would I recognize it if I had it?

It is difficult to say what the 'usual' symptoms of MS are, in the sense of those being experienced uniformly by everyone with the condition. Indeed, one of the characteristics of MS is the variability of symptoms, that result from the many different parts of the nervous system affected by the condition. In the early stages of the disease there are no exclusive 'MS symptoms' that define a diagnosis of MS, because all of the most frequent symptoms associated with it can also be caused individually by other conditions, and these must be ruled out before a diagnosis of MS can be made.

Nevertheless, there are some more common symptoms, experienced in different combinations and to different degrees by people in the early stages of MS, that might indicate that MS is one possible cause:

- **Sensory symptoms** – these can occasionally be dramatic, such as:
  - temporary visual disturbances (including double or blurred vision) or even temporary loss of sight;

- frequent or continuing tingling sensations and numbness without other good cause.

• **Muscular coordination problems:**

  - muscular weakness (known medically as paresis);

  - poor coordination and balance;

  - tightening or rigidity in particular muscle groups (known medically as spasticity);

  - more infrequently, temporary paralysis of certain muscle groups.

• **Bladder, bowel and sexual function** problems may sometimes occur in the very early stages of the disease.

• **Unusual forgetfulness, disorientation, confusion** and (very, very rarely) **fits** or **seizures** occur occasionally with the onset of MS.

This range of possible symptoms of MS is very large, and every one can be caused by other conditions, many of which are not serious. Furthermore the symptoms, especially in the early stages of MS, may vary from day to day or even from hour to hour in any one person and, as we have noted, may also vary greatly between different individuals. People in the early stages of MS may experience just one, or several of them.

Many of the early symptoms of MS, especially if their onset is gradual, are difficult even for the people themselves to distinguish and describe precisely, although they may feel that something is wrong with them. Thus the point at which people seek the advice of others, and particularly medical advice, can be very variable.

I have symptoms which are like those described for MS in my health encyclopedia. I know something is wrong, but I am afraid of being diagnosed with MS. What should I do?

In general it is better to know what's wrong with you, than to continue to be anxious and worried. Research with people who subsequently turned out to have MS has shown that some had thought that they had conditions which, in their terms, would have been far worse, such as a brain tumour, or indeed that they were 'going mad', because of the varied and unusual nature of their symptoms. Some were quite relieved when they knew they had MS. Most people like to have a medical explanation of increasingly puzzling symptoms, especially those which may upset their daily routines. In any case – if it is MS – the symptoms will not go away permanently, even if they do so temporarily; getting help and information from medical or health care staff; from other people with the condition, or from organizations like the MS Society, can be a great support.

I have heard people talk about 'attacks' of MS. What does that mean?

Symptoms of MS often appear quite suddenly, although they may be relatively mild early in the disease, as the protective myelin sheath of the nerve concerned is damaged so much (see Chapter 1) that the transmission of messages to the muscles or sensory organs is interrupted. Sometimes this process affects one set of nerves, and sometimes it affects several sets. Such a process, whether general or more specific, is often called 'an episode', 'an attack' or, when it recurs, 'an exacerbation', 'a relapse' or 'a flare-up' of MS. Symptoms may almost disappear as some repair of the myelin takes place, particularly early in the disease, and 'inflammation' or swelling around the damaged areas subsides over the course of a few minutes, hours or sometimes days. When such symptoms disappear or become less severe, this process is usually called 'a remission'. However, there is always likely to be some residual damage to the nerves involved. Thus the same symptom is likely to reappear again, but this may not be for days, weeks, months, and sometimes for many years. As the disease progresses, damage will occur at new nerve sites and, from time to time, new symptoms will appear.

Some people have one or two attacks or relapses and then there are no further symptoms for many years. At the other extreme some people may experience almost continuous progression without any distinct remissions or attacks, but just a general decline in either sensory or muscle control, or both. In between these two extremes is the most frequent pattern of MS, consisting of shorter periods of attacks or relapses, separated by longer periods of gradual recovery, i.e. remissions.

What sort of symptoms will I start to experience now that I have been diagnosed with MS?

Being given a diagnosis of MS does not in itself mean that you will experience any more symptoms than you did before. It is possible that you will feel more conscious of 'MS-type symptoms' now, perhaps because you have read or thought about them more, or had discussions with your doctor or others about them. However, if you mean will you experience the same, and perhaps other, symptoms as time passes following the diagnosis, then the answer is probably yes for most people. MS is known as a *progressive neurological disease*, even though we are still not good at predicting when, how and in what ways it will progress. Most people will experience a recurrence of the same symptoms that they had before, although the degree and the timing of that recurrence is difficult to judge precisely. From time to time, new symptoms will probably appear, as the course of the disease affects another nerve pathway. It is hard to say what those new symptoms will actually be in any individual. They may be linked in some way to those you have already experienced, but completely new sensory or *motor* (movement-related) *symptoms* may appear.

It is important, however, not to be constantly preoccupied in waiting for a new symptom to appear. It may occur in weeks or months, but you may be one of the more fortunate people with MS who never has another new symptom.

What will the course of my MS be?

As we have stressed, the most frustrating aspect of MS for everybody concerned is the high degree of individual variation in symptoms, and the unpredictable speed of individual progression of the disease. Thus with present knowledge, it is impossible to predict the exact future course of the condition in any one person at the time of diagnosis. A great deal of systematic and detailed research is now being undertaken on tracing how the disease develops over many years in large numbers of people with MS. In due course this research should assist doctors to give more accurate information earlier.

The full range of **possible** disease courses following diagnosis can, in principle, be very large, from almost no further symptoms on the one hand, to a relatively quick progression to serious disability on the other. As a very rough guide, at any one time about one-third of all people with MS appear to be experiencing no serious relapses, about one-third are having a distinct relapsing-remitting course with relapses of varying severity, and about one-third are experiencing a chronically progressive course. About one-third of all people with MS have serious disabilities and require significant everyday support, and a further third require what might be described as significant lifestyle adjustments to manage their lives with MS.

I have just been diagnosed with MS, after waiting about 11 months for a diagnosis. I don't feel any worse than when I first went to the doctor. How soon will I be in a wheelchair?

In general the progression of MS is slowest, and the outlook (often called the *prognosis*), is best for people who are diagnosed under the age of 40, and who have an initial relapsing-remitting history. However, the long-term prognosis, even in these cases, is impossible to predict with any certainty. A rather more helpful – although not entirely accurate – prediction can be made after assessing your disease for five years or so, taking into account the number as well as the severity of relapses over this period, and comparing your symptoms now with those five years previously. The working basis of the 'five-year rule', as it is sometimes referred to, is that what has happened to you in the first five years will be a reasonable guide to what is going to happen in the medium term. Even this rule cannot be considered by any means infallible. It is just a guide.

For you, even after waiting 11 months – which seems a long time – the prognosis cannot be determined with any great accuracy. However, we can look positively at the situation: from recent research only about one-fifth of people with MS appear to be seriously disabled, to the extent of requiring major assistance (such as a wheelchair) for their mobility, within 15 years following their diagnosis.

Just as an important aside at this point, many people – certainly when they are first diagnosed, or indeed when they suspect they have MS – think of being in a wheelchair as the thing they most fear about the disease, and what they most wish to avoid (see the section on *Chairs and wheelchairs* in Chapter 10). This is, in part, because of the premium our society places on being independent and mobile, and the ways in which people in wheelchairs have been treated in the past. Moreover, it is always difficult to picture yourself in the future, in a situation when you have less of something than you have now, but this will happen to all of us at some point, whether we have MS or not. The experience of life is that almost all of us adapt to such situations pretty well when they occur, even though in prospect they may be rather forbidding. In any case, as far as both coping with mobility and the public perception of people in wheelchairs go, there is a positive sea change taking place.

I know that many symptoms are linked to MS. Are there any particular ones which might catch me by surprise?

Many people with MS feel that almost all of their symptoms surprise them! Indeed it is a characteristic of the disease that you may be taken unawares by a symptom, as MS often develops in unpredictable ways. However, at any one time, you will gradually attune yourself to the way that your body now works with MS, and what might be described as your 'normal' symptoms in life with the disease – although you do have to be prepared for such symptoms to vary from day to day. Two kinds of symptoms stand out particularly as ones which people with MS frequently say are surprising, not so much because they exist, but because of how they affect many aspects of life:

- The first set of symptoms are those related to **fatigue**. Lots of people with MS complain that, on occasions, and sometimes more regularly, they feel extraordinarily tired – much more so than with anything else, even looking after children! This tiredness, which is usually described as MS fatigue, is something which people with MS say is both very unpredictable, and difficult to manage, so they have to pace themselves carefully and be prepared to adapt their lives from day to day, even hour to hour. We explore some of the reasons for such fatigue and ways of managing it in Chapter 9.

- The second set of symptoms is to do with what doctors often refer to colloquially as your **waterworks**, i.e. to do with your bladder and urination. Many people with MS, perhaps 75–90%, do have some problems of this kind, although the nature of these problems differs widely. Early on in the disease there may be very few difficulties: a little more *urgency* perhaps, i.e. wanting to urinate more suddenly and possibly more often, or having some problems over control, e.g. unexpectedly leaking a little. Whilst these particular problems may be considered medically to be modest or minor, for people with MS they may involve quite a lot of thought and careful planning. Much later in the disease process these problems can become substantial, and require several strategies to manage them (discussed in Chapter 7). An important point concerning all bladder problems associated with MS is that some recent studies have found a high proportion of those with urinary problems also have bladder infections that may exacerbate those problems considerably, as well as possibly causing pain. Such infections can be cured, in most cases, with appropriate antibiotic treatment. So get help from your doctor on this issue and don't just assume that all your difficulties with your bladder are caused directly by the MS itself.

Overall, the issue of unpredictability could probably be regarded as the most surprising characteristic of many symptoms of MS, particularly in terms of managing your life from day to day.

Can you die from MS and if so, how does it kill you, and how soon?

MS is not considered a fatal disease in itself. You are almost as likely to die from a cause which is unrelated to MS (e.g. heart disease) as one associated with the effects of the disease. As far as MS itself is concerned, over considerable time, **if the symptoms of the disease become very severe** (and for the vast majority of people with the disease, this is many years, and almost certainly decades ahead), they may affect a number of other body systems which can lead to death. Such consequences could be described medically as very serious *sequelae* of the disease. Severely reduced mobility over long periods of time, in conjunction with the effects of MS on the control of breathing, swallowing and kidney function, can precipitate conditions (such as pneumonia or serious blood or kidney infections) that could lead to death. However, these possible causes of death are well known to those who provide specialist care for people with MS, and thus preventative action can often be taken well in advance to minimize the risk of death.

On a more optimistic note, although people with MS face more causes of death compared to other people, their life expectancy now is encouragingly close to that of the population at large. It is also encouraging that, since the 1960s, because it has improved from a previously lower initial figure, the increase in life expectancy of people with MS has been faster than that of the general population. This suggests that the health care of people with severe MS, amongst other factors, has been more effective at reducing premature deaths.

3
The causes of MS

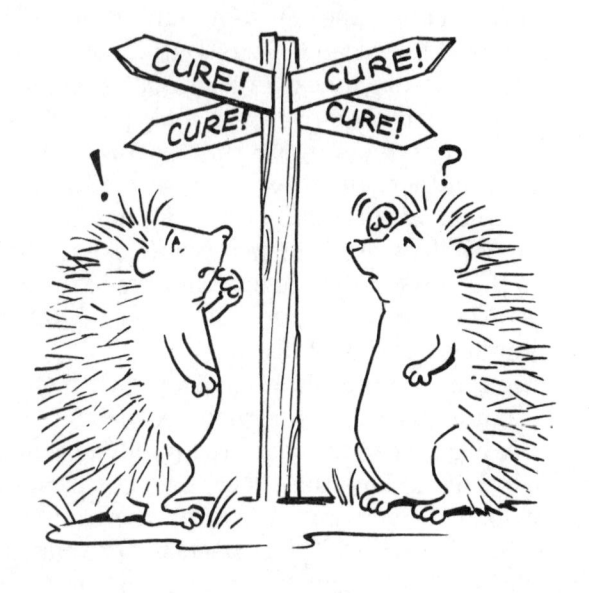

The cause or causes of MS are still unknown. Although there are significant geographical variations in the distribution of people with MS throughout the world, a great deal of research effort has failed to uncover any tangible evidence that there are any specific avoidable risk factors associated with the onset of the disease. Despite these points, internal changes in the body, and particularly in the central nervous system that are involved in the onset and progression of the disease, have been studied in great detail, and there are therapies designed to lessen the effects of all of the most serious symptoms of the condition.

At present, the most likely cause appears to be a combination of genetic and environmental factors. Studies of identical twins, where one or both has MS, offer what might be called the 'purest' way in which to investigate this theory: it appears that genetic factors contribute between 30 and 35% and environmental factors about 65–70% of the total contribution to the cause. These two figures suggest that further research needs to be undertaken on both issues. There does not seem to be one simple gene linked to MS.

Environmentally, many different factors could be involved; furthermore, the precise relationship between environmental and genetic factors is very unclear. Despite the speed of research, particularly on the study of genetic factors, findings from these studies which may help to control the onset or management of MS will not be available for several years.

Media hype

Almost every week I read in the newspaper, or hear on the television, reports of scientists claiming to have discovered the 'cause' and the 'cure' of MS. No sooner has such a claim been made, than there is another completely contradictory one. Yet I still seem to be no nearer getting my MS cured.

One of the biggest concerns of many people with MS is the almost constant trickle, and occasionally flood, of news stories announcing that very significant progress has been made towards establishing the 'cause' or a 'cure' for MS. Such claims in the past have turned out to be, at best, very premature – in effect announcing a small amount of progress along a very, very long road; at worst they are false in the sense of being misleading, not only about the extent, but also the direction of progress.

However, it is important to say that the most reputable and likely way in which the cause(s) of MS will be uncovered is through the gradual and systematic application of scientific research. Mostly, such research moves slowly and cautiously, building on previous findings. Only rarely is there 'a breakthrough' in the sense that people with MS understand the word. However, to scientists who have been struggling with the complicated jigsaw puzzle of MS for years, even a small step can be considered a 'breakthrough', allowing them to proceed to the next stage of the puzzle. We discuss research into MS more thoroughly in Chapter 17.

First, research, by definition, is about the unknown, and is bound to lead to contradictory claims, as scientists in different disciplines and with different ideas come up with different ways of understanding a disease such as MS. Each of these must be subjected to rigorous review and confirmation. Secondly, researchers, like everyone else, are frankly under pressure to promote their own work, to develop their careers, and gain funds and other resources to continue their research. Thirdly, journalists rarely understand the subject fully and are under pressure to generate exciting news items – this is usually where announcements of finding the cause, or the cure, usually appear.

Don't be misled by newspaper and television reports. MS research (and much of medical science) is a complicated subject and cannot be condensed into a brief news report. If a breakthrough really does occur from one group of scientists, then it will need to be replicated, by other researchers, to check out such claims. As a 'rule of thumb', a breakthrough is worth taking more seriously once three or more research groups have independently confirmed similar findings. In any case such a cure, even if it came, would require several years of testing before it became readily available to people with MS.

Genetics

If MS is at least partly genetic, are my children going to have MS?

It has been known from very early studies on MS that there is a *familial component* to the disease, especially in relation to a small proportion of families where more than one person has, or has had MS. This familial component is now known to be at least partly genetic, rather than purely the result of a shared environment or similarities in lifestyle between family members. However, the inheritance pattern of MS is complicated; it is not easily predicted, as it is for muscular dystrophy or red hair, for example, where there is a single gene which can be traced through 'family trees' (often called *family pedigrees* in genetic research).

The risk of having MS in the population as a whole is about 1 in 1000 over a lifetime. This risk has been calculated at about 5% or 1 in 20 for a first-degree blood relative of someone with MS (e.g. a child or a brother or sister), and is still very small compared to many of the more significant risks that we all run. To look at it another way there is a 95% chance that your child will not subsequently have MS. The risk, however, for an identical twin of a person with MS (i.e. someone who shares exactly the same genetic material) is about 200 times higher, or approaching 1 in 3, although this risk still indicates that only one twin is affected by MS in most (67%) pairs of identical twins with the genetic susceptibility. At present it is not possible to tell prenatally whether any one child is more at risk than any other.

Is there a genetic test for MS, or for the risk of MS, as a result of the discoveries in genetics?

No, not at the moment, but it is a very real possibility for the future. When researchers have found the combination of genes associated with a susceptibility to MS in one or other forms then, in principle, a test could be developed with the use of a small blood sample.

As researchers increasingly unravel many genetic links to various diseases, then tests can be quickly devised to indicate the presence of a relevant gene, or a combination of genes. However, even if such a test proves positive, it is unlikely that anything could be done directly to alter the genetic make-up of any individual for several years or even decades, and probably not before MS actually occurs. The lesson of genetic research in relation to cystic fibrosis is salutary: it was thought 10 years ago that routine gene therapy would be quickly available for this condition which has a relatively simple genetic cause, but in fact such therapy has taken far longer.

In the future, tests might indicate people who have a genetic make-up making them susceptible to MS, indicating that they might have, say, a 30% chance of developing the disease by the age of 50. The issue then becomes, would they want to know? What would they do if they did know? Would other family members want to know? Would insurance companies, or employers be able to exert pressure for such a test, and make important decisions about your lifestyle as a result? The implications of both having and using such a test must be thought through very carefully so that sensible and ethical judgements about how to proceed can be made. At the very least, substantial professional support needs to be available to those who might take such tests.

Five of my relatives, over three generations, have had MS. Are we a family with a special risk of MS?

There are a number of issues here. There is known to be an enhanced risk for 'blood-related' family members, once a member is recognized as having had MS, and particularly an enhanced risk for brothers/sisters and children. Thus it would not be surprising if more than one person in a family did have MS, given the relatively large number of people worldwide who have the disease. Of course, complete coincidences occur as well, where two family members unrelated by blood have MS. However, your family (or some of its members) may unfortunately have an unusually potent genetic susceptibility to MS. The only consolation here is that families such as yours seem to acquire a form of the disease with early onset, but generally with slower rates of progression than others. The current fast pace of work on the genetics of MS will probably pinpoint the special susceptibilities in families like yours relatively soon. However, there is another point. Looking back it is often difficult to be clear about a diagnosis of MS, of course. You may well be right that all your relatives stretching back several generations have had MS, but because diagnostic techniques are now more refined, it is sometimes difficult to be sure retrospectively.

Connections with other diseases

When I had an infection last year, my MS suddenly flared up. The attack was particularly bad and I still haven't fully recovered. Could this have been a cause of the disease in the first place? If the attack was caused by the infection, should I avoid people and places where I might catch something?

There is no conclusive evidence of a link between either a particular bacterial or viral infection and the onset or 'flare-up' of MS, although this is, in fact, quite commonly reported. Such a link is more likely to be repeated during the course – rather than before the onset – of the disease. It is possible that the link you describe is coincidence, although recent research is uncovering a range of associations between a damaged immune system, infections and 'exacerbations' or 'flare-ups' in MS.

If your general health is reasonable, then the chances of anything affecting your MS further are decreased. Practically, it is not usually possible to 'avoid people and places', and how we 'catch' infections is complicated. It depends as much on our own state of health as the presence of 'germs' or 'infections' in other people. In fact most of us have many 'germs' already in or on our own bodies which could make us ill, but their effects are only triggered by combinations of many circumstances.

I have read that at least some cases of MS are directly caused by infection with a herpes virus, HHV-6. Is this true?

There has been much research on infections of the nervous system, and their association with MS. However, for a link with MS to be confirmed, a higher incidence of the particular infection has to be found in people with MS than in people without MS, as well as a far lower rate of MS in people without the infection. Over many years, no virus has yet met these two criteria consistently, although occasionally (as now, in the case of the herpes

virus HHV-6), a new candidate appears that seems to offer a
promising line of investigation.

Even if an association had been confirmed, it still would not
prove that the infection was the cause of the MS. MS is a dysfunction of the immune system and the MS itself may already
make it more likely that people with the disease will be infected
with a range of viruses, rather than the virus itself being the
cause of the MS.

**I have heard a lot about Lyme's disease recently. Can that
cause MS?**
No. There is no evidence that Lyme's disease causes MS, but it
can be mistaken for MS in the early stages of diagnosis. Lyme's
disease is a bacterial infection, usually transmitted by ticks. It is
a potentially serious condition, and can have a range of neurological effects, some of which seem close to some symptoms of
MS. The bacterium which causes this infection, whose grand
name is *Borrelia burgdorferii*, is endemic amongst wild deer
and various other animals, who often harbour ticks and other
blood-sucking parasites. A bite from a tick carrying infected
blood from a wild animal can transmit the infection to humans.
The New Forest in England, in particular, and some parts of the
United States are affected, and walkers should wear sensible
protection against tick bites, just as they would to protect themselves against mosquitoes. The good thing is, once recognized,
Lyme's disease can be successfully treated with a long course of
high-dose antibiotics. A complex blood test can confirm the possibility of this particular bacterial or viral infection.

**Someone at my MS support group claims that MS can be
caused by several bacterial infections, and I have been
treated recently for a candidal infection. Is there a link?**

Research has not shown MS to be caused by any particular bacterial infection; however, it is possible that the timing of a
relapse may coincide with a bacterial or viral infection. This
could be due to a change in immune activity which allows the

infection to gain hold: the bacterial infection can trigger an immune response, or both the relapse and the infection may occur in response to some unknown third factor.

At present there is a widespread interest, particularly amongst many involved in alternative or complementary medicine, in *Candida albicans* (thrush). Although candida can be associated with many symptoms, as well as having a low-level but debilitating effect on health, there is almost no formal evidence that it is associated with relapses of MS in itself. The reason for the existence of candidal infection is also a matter of debate: it may be a result rather than a cause of a weakened immune system, and it is also known to be more common as a side effect of some anti-inflammatory drugs used in MS. Of course, any infection with potentially problematic symptoms should be treated with topical antibiotics.

I have recently read that influenza injections, which are promoted at my doctor's practice, can make MS much worse. Should I avoid having a 'flu jab, or take the doctor's advice and have one?

Many people with MS naturally look for a preceding event to explain why their symptoms have worsened, or why they have had an 'attack' or 'relapse'. One of the most obvious events is an injection, not least because most people remember such an event, for few of us enjoy it! However, research studies have failed to demonstrate any link between the injections (vaccinations or inoculations) and any subsequent worsening of the MS. Nevertheless, other factors going on in your life at the time of the injection, but not the injection itself, might have been linked with the subsequent course of your MS. Fatigue, and possibly what we call 'stress', could have had some effect. However, although most people with MS probably feel that undue stress in their lives may bring on a relapse, scientifically this issue is still being argued over. Even so, many people have their own ideas about things that they feel are linked with their MS symptoms, and try to avoid them.

Is MS associated in any way with other diseases?

The answer is generally no – in the sense that MS is not **known** to be caused by them, although retrospectively many people with MS can point to symptoms and illnesses which seem to have preceded its onset. Research on the patterns of MS in the community is going on and discussed in Chapter 17.

Of course as MS progresses, it may itself give rise, in effect, to other conditions, through a weakened immune system, for example. Respiratory and urinary infections are amongst the most common problems when MS becomes more serious. Almost all of these can be cured, if treated promptly. Occasionally, other unrelated conditions might affect you, especially as you get older.

Is MS linked with cancer, which also runs in my family?

No. There is no known link between cancer of any type and MS. However, as cancer constitutes one of the leading causes of death in the Western world, accounting for over a quarter of all deaths, it is to be expected that some people with MS will also develop cancer, but no more frequently than people who haven't. As the possibility of developing most forms of cancer increases with age, reaching a peak as people reach their late 60s, and as the life expectancy of people with MS increases, so these coincidences may become slightly more common. However, we repeat that cancer is no more, and no less likely in families affected by MS, than it is in other families.

Is MS a different and more severe form of another autoimmune disease, such as lupus or arthritis?

There are strong similarities between some aspects of these conditions and some aspects of MS. All these diseases are considered to be autoimmune disorders where the immune system is triggered into mistakenly attacking normal tissues in the body and causing repeated inflammation and damage. Whilst traditionally a lot of research has been disease-specific, where scientists become 'MS researchers' or 'arthritis researchers', there has been renewed interest in how the immune system works and the broader processes at work in all these conditions. Because there are still very substantial differences in the age and gender composition of the people who are affected, more specific explanations will always be needed as to why a particular disease develops. At present these conditions are still thought to be completely separate disease entities.

I broke my arm a few weeks before the first symptoms of my MS started. Do you think that could possibly have caused my MS?

The relationship of 'trauma' or 'traumatic injuries' to MS has been studied for several years. Many people with MS have reported accidents or injuries in the weeks or months before the onset of MS or occurrence of relapses. Studies have compared people with and without MS for the incidence of head injuries, sprains, major and minor surgery, burns, dental work, fractures, abrasions and bruises. Accident and injury rates have been compared in people with MS who have had relapses and those who have not. Almost all the studies have concluded that there is no significant difference in numbers, or in the effect of trauma in causing or worsening MS, although a few researchers still believe in some relationship of trauma to the progression of MS.

Even so, doesn't it make sense that a head injury, or an injury near the brain or spinal cord, might have some effect on MS? After all, isn't it the central nervous system which is the main thing damaged in MS?

Head injuries and their relationship to the onset or course of MS have been widely studied, but very little evidence of such a link (as with other injuries) has been found. A more general issue is whether such injuries may have broken what is called the *blood–brain barrier* (in short the BBB). Normally the brain is 'insulated' from direct contact with blood. In other words, blood necessarily circulates around brain tissue, but never comes into contact with it directly. Some scientists have argued that when this barrier is broken – through injury or through some internal damage – some parts of the CNS may themselves become contaminated and thus be damaged by the various blood products that are released. In the 1980s a small minority of doctors believed that MS might be produced and exacerbated by such a contamination; this led to the view that a particular therapy – treatment by hyperbaric (high pressure) oxygen (HBO) – might lessen the damage (see Chapter 6). This particular blood system-related theory of MS and other neurological conditions and the treatment is widely disputed, and still a matter of lively debate. There continues to be both advocacy and availability of HBO therapy in many MS Therapy Centres in Britain which were established under the former national organization Action for Research into Multiple Sclerosis (ARMS).

Environmental

You mentioned possible environmental causes of MS earlier. What are they?

When we talk about possible environmental causes of MS, it really means almost everything that is not a genetic or inherited cause – such as heavy metal poisoning; injuries or trauma; illness; climate; diet; food allergies. Perhaps one of the problems is that people with MS and scientists looked and hoped for some simple environmental substance, problem or illness that might by itself cause MS; this would have led to an antidote and to other people in the future being able to avoid the disease. In fact, as we noted earlier, it is almost certain that MS is caused by a combination of genetic susceptibility (in other words, inherited characteristics) and environmental, i.e. non-genetic, factors. It is also possible that several environmental factors may be involved and thus, unfortunately, the search for a single environmental cause of MS may be a much too simple a view of how the disease arises.

I have heard that MS is caused by chronic lead or mercury poisoning, so why aren't the doctors doing more to warn people about the dangers of dental fillings containing mercury?

It is certainly true that an excess of some heavy metals in the body such as lead, mercury and cadmium, may result in serious neurological damage, and thus in recognizable neurological symptoms. There are well documented cases of both individuals and groups of people in geographical 'clusters', who have had 'MS-like' symptoms after (usually) major industrial/occupational exposure to one or more heavy metals. Lead in particular is a prominent cause of neurological damage and is gradually disappearing from our environment as lead waterpipes, lead-based paints and lead petrol additives are replaced with safer alternatives. However, although both excess lead and MS lead to neurological damage, there is no evidence that excess lead causes MS.

As regards mercury-based fillings in teeth, there are two separate issues here, one of which is whether the fillings may have produced neurological symptoms in people who have (perhaps mistakenly) been diagnosed with MS. The other is whether mercury fillings may have caused MS itself, or at least made it worse. It should be said that there is a veritable mountain of research and opinion on both sides of the argument. As we have already stated, there is no doubt that excess mercury can produce neurological damage; thus the issues are how much mercury has been released into the body through these dental fillings, what mechanisms might have led to particular damage to an individual's nervous system, and what relationship this damage has to the onset or course of MS. A fundamental difficulty for those who support the mercury fillings/MS argument is that a large proportion of the adult population will have had at least some mercury fillings in their lifetimes, and yet only a fraction of those people have MS.

There may be a few people with a special sensitivity to mercury who develop MS, when others have not, but this is a matter of further detailed scientific research. Dental amalgam does contain mercury which can erode over time and be absorbed into the blood stream. However, this is a very small contribution to the amount of mercury ingested by most people (deep-sea fish is a much greater source), and the exposure to dental amalgam is well within the safety limits currently recommended for mercury.

In the meantime, some people with MS are having their mercury fillings removed and replaced by composite fillings (which do not contain mercury). This is a costly, time-consuming and painful process, and actually results in greater initial mercury exposure (when the old fillings are removed by drilling) than if the fillings were left unreplaced – unless extraordinary precautions are taken. If you do feel that mercury dental amalgam is a major issue for you, then a safer alternative is probably to ask that all fillings are replaced by composite material, but only as and when those mercury-based fillings need replacing anyway. However, this must be your personal decision at present, for the majority of scientific opinion is that there is little or no direct relationship between mercury fillings and the onset or course of MS.

Diet

The whole subject of diet and nutrition is discussed at greater length in Chapter 11. Here the controversial issue of whether diet might 'cause' MS is considered.

Is it possible that a 'bad diet' might cause MS?

This is an argument often to do with the effects of some of the 'bad' elements in contemporary Western diets, such as excess saturated fats (e.g. those contained in many animal and dairy products) which appear to have detrimental effects on general health. The particular role that they might play in relation to MS symptoms or in counteracting the positive role of *essential fatty acids* (see Chapter 11), which are 'good' as opposed to 'bad' substances, is now under discussion. Many no- or low-saturated fat diets have been devised, often by people with MS themselves or their relatives, which have been claimed by some to improve their MS. Indeed, there is some scientific but still disputed evidence to support the view that a low-saturated fat diet might reduce the number, or severity, of relapses for some people, or perhaps even slow the course of the disease in others.

Another related argument is one that has focused on the role of poor diets, especially those which might be deficient in the essential fatty acids mentioned above. However, if such diets led to MS, then we would expect many more cases of the disease and its distribution to be very different, in particular amongst the many populations in the world living in famine conditions or with very poor nutrition. Researchers have pointed out that one of the other characteristics of the world distribution of MS is that the disease is far more common in temperate countries where relatively high levels of saturated fats, meat and dairy produce are consumed, and so it may not be a poor diet (low calorie and low protein) in itself which is the problem, but more the imbalances between 'good' and 'bad' fat intake. In either case, if it was just diet that was concerned, we would expect far more cases of MS, and it seems very likely that MS is linked to some defective mechanism in particular people which causes less of the essential fatty acids to be employed in building or maintaining nervous system tissue, and thus leads to the broader symptoms and signs of MS in due course.

Nevertheless, a low-saturated fat diet is recommended by many health educators as being the best kind of diet for general health, and on these grounds alone could benefit people with MS.

I have heard that food allergy may be to blame for MS. What are your thoughts on that?

There is almost no formal scientific evidence to support this view, but many people with or without MS think that there are an increasing number of food allergies associated with many different illnesses, symptoms or reactions. You will have to decide for yourself whether any particular diet you wish to pursue is too inconvenient or costly in terms of what you feel you might gain from it. (One of the most widely known and used is a 'gluten-free' diet.) There is more about this in the Section on *Diet and nutrition* in Chapter 11.

The overall position as regards diet and MS is:

- There has been less research on diet and MS than on other aspects of the disease.

- There are good grounds for saying that diet is likely to have some bearing in the medium and longer term on general health and perhaps, through that, on the ways in which people manage their MS.

- There is little evidence that any particular diet has major effects on the course of MS, but some evidence suggests that a low-saturated fat diet may be beneficial for some people in relation to relapses.

- Finally, there is little or no evidence that poor diet in itself causes MS – if this were so, the geographic and social distribution of MS would be very different.

Why me? Can it be my fault?

I know that some people get MS, but why has it happened to me?

Perhaps the question most often asked by people with MS or, of course, with other serious medical conditions, is 'Why me?' It is the most obvious question, and yet the most difficult to answer. There are a number of reasons, speaking scientifically, why this should be so.

First, because we do not know the precise cause(s) of MS, it is difficult to identify the risk factors that might give rise to the onset of the disease, whether you yourself had some or all of them, and thus whether you were at risk or not. Secondly, even if we did know all the risk factors, we might still not be able to predict accurately that you either would or would not have developed MS. Most risk factors, even if put all together, still only suggest probabilities, not certainties for one individual. Thirdly, even in situations where we know the exact cause of a disease, such as a specific infection like influenza, as well as most of the risk factors, there are often other elusive factors which seem to mean that one person has the 'flu rather than someone else, even though the two people seem similar in almost all other respects. In principle, therefore, although scientists believe that, given time and resources, all the factors which give rise to MS in particular individuals will be identified, problems in predicting such individual outcomes with other 'simpler' diseases indicate that this may be an ambitious goal in the short term.

I know it sounds silly, but I often feel that I've been punished in having MS, for some bad things that I did earlier in my life. I know it's not true, but I keep feeling like this.

Because of the difficulty in identifying scientifically who will develop MS, many other personal explanations arise. Although often it is too difficult to talk about easily with others, people may feel that their MS is, as it were, a punishment for some wrong that they have done in the past, or is in some other way a moral judgement on them. Everyone needs to place things that happen to them in the context of what might be described as their own 'meaning of life', and this often has a moral dimension. However, apart from all the other information we have about the specific causes of MS, there is, of course, no evidence that people with MS are morally worse (or indeed any better) than anyone else, nor that diseases only occur in people who have done 'bad things'. Many 'saint-like' people have diseases that are difficult to manage. Scientists and almost every doctor believe that disease does not result in any sense from any kind of moral wrongdoing; they can therefore be very reassuring on this particular issue. If these particular concerns continue to worry you and affect other areas of your life, you could seek advice and support from your GP.

My first symptoms of MS started when I was working hard for a promotion at work and exhausting myself on a daily basis. Could I have avoided MS by slowing down a bit back then?

Almost certainly not. Increasing evidence from the study of the development of MS suggests that it starts to occur – in terms of its onset and the beginning of damage to the myelin (see Chapter 1) – over many months, if not many years, probably well before the first symptoms become evident. Your point also suggests that we know the cause of MS, which we do not. However, it is natural and tempting to associate a major life event, or a difficult period in one's life, with a disease like MS. It is possible that, when the symptoms occurred, they became immediately more recognizable, and indeed may have had a more significant effect on your life, because you were working so hard with little room to manoeuvre.

I have MS and I am gay, but my brother, who isn't gay, is completely healthy. Is there some kind of link between being gay and MS?

No! Most people affected by a dramatic change, such as developing MS, try to find some event, or other factor to blame. There is no evidence that being gay has anything to do with you having MS or, conversely, that being heterosexual offers any protection from the disease at all. It is simply a coincidence.

A more general point, raised by your question, is what we might describe as *selective recall*. This affects many retrospective studies seeking to find factors associated with the onset of MS. People with MS often have good reason to recall some part or event in their lives which has great meaning to them, but not to recall others that may, from a researcher's point of view, be equally or much more important in the attempt to ascertain possible causes of the disease. This *recall bias* can result in what proves to be a false association between earlier events and the onset of MS.

I have always been teetotal, a non-smoker, have eaten well, and kept as fit as a I could, but I have MS. I know some people who have no respect for their health, smoke too much, eat unhealthy diets (and one is even an alcoholic) – but they seem perfectly OK. Why did I get MS?

The point you make is, of course, one of the paradoxes of life: many of us believe that, if we follow all the available advice about healthy living (not smoking, drinking moderately, doing regular exercise, eating a healthy diet), we shall not fall ill, and certainly not get a serious disease like MS. However, such advice is only about probabilities. In other words, in a large population of people and all other things being equal, if everyone followed these 'health rules', more of that population would live longer and with less illness. But all other things are not equal. There are many other risk factors that come into play for particular individuals, including their inherited make-up, which they can do little to change at present. It is some of these other factors, despite your strenuous attempts to live a healthy life, that may well have come into play in your case. Conversely, there may be similar protective (rather than risk) factors that operate in the case of a few people who are living unhealthy lifestyles which means that they can still keep healthy. So, although individually we cannot be certain that healthy lifestyles will protect you from illness, you will certainly have more chances of staying healthy.

4
Diagnosing MS

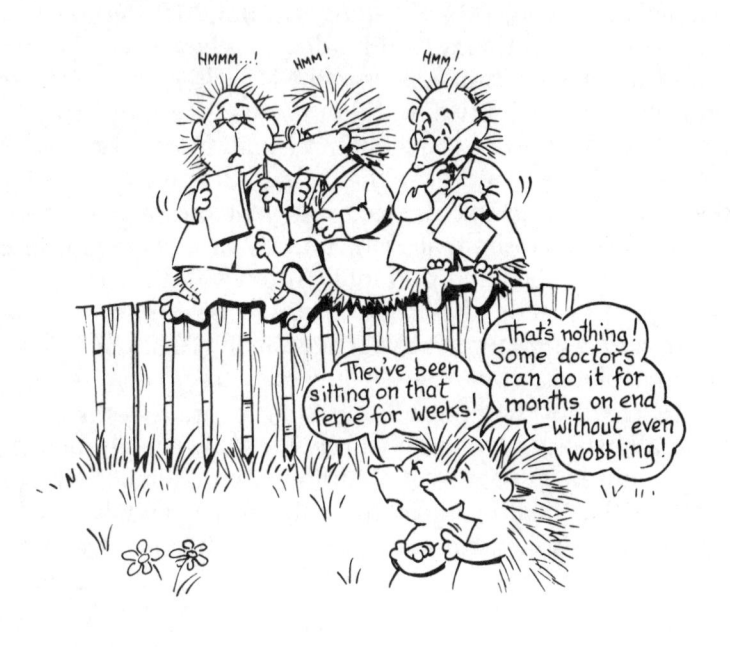

The diagnosis of MS has always been a long, slow and complicated process. There is no definitive laboratory test for MS. Even some of the newer and sophisticated brain scanning techniques that are beginning to be more widely used, such as nuclear magnetic resonance (NMR) scanning which can locate lesions or patchy scarring (scleroses) in the nervous system, require very careful interpretation by a skilled doctor. In addition, many people in the early stages of MS do not exhibit the 'classic' symptoms and laboratory signs that are considered to be the 'textbook'

features of the disease. Finally, many other conditions may produce symptoms almost indistinguishable from MS symptoms. Thus the complexity in diagnosing MS lies in establishing sufficient evidence to establish a diagnosis of MS beyond reasonable doubt by excluding other possibilities.

How will I know?

I think I might have symptoms of MS. How do I know whether I have the disease or not?

This is a question which can really only be answered after a detailed investigation by a neurologist, i.e. the medical specialist who deals with problems affecting the central nervous system (CNS). It cannot be definitively answered by a general practitioner (GP) without access to further tests undertaken by a neurologist, and an answer should not be assumed from just consulting a book such as this.

This question is sometimes asked by people, who may have read or heard about MS, or know someone with MS, and then feel that they may have symptoms that are compatible with a diagnosis of MS. The nature of the disease – the variability in its associated symptoms and the way they often appear to come and go – encourages this view. You need to remember, however, that every single one of the symptoms associated with MS can be caused by other conditions. It is your particular pattern of symptoms over time, together with additional signs – objective and standardized medical assessments – which are used to make a diagnosis. Thus, if you are concerned, you should initially seek the advice of your GP.

Of course, you may have already consulted your GP about your symptoms. Although we keep stressing this, it is likely that, apart from when the symptoms are unusually dramatic, your doctor may initially pursue a strategy of what has been described as 'watchful waiting'; others have called it 'the investigation of time'. In other words, your doctor will see how your symptoms develop, and whether they return or not – at least to eliminate other minor or temporary causes of those symptoms. This may be a frustrating time for you, as you may feel that you are not getting a clear and immediate answer to your problems. The GP may also think that your presenting symptoms are not to do with problems in the CNS. Many symptoms of MS could be caused by difficulties in other body systems, and thus initially may not be treated as neurological symptoms. If you are concerned and anxious about your symptoms, and do not feel that the GP is making as much progress as you wish in tracking down their cause, there is no reason why you should not ask for a second or specialist opinion.

How is MS usually diagnosed?

Sometimes, a person, who already has a clear history of a first 'attack' and then several 'relapses' with remissions over time, and with identifiable MS symptoms in each case that fit the 'classic' pattern of the disease, might consult their GP and then be referred fairly rapidly to a neurologist. In such a situation, a neurologist may be able, at least in principle, to make a formal clinical diagnosis relatively quickly, once confirming signs have been established by examination, and perhaps one or two other tests have been undertaken. However, more often symptoms are less clear cut – more an awareness that something is wrong than anything very specific that could immediately be attributed to MS – and the diagnosis can then be a long drawn-out process.

Although the criteria by which neurologists diagnose the disease is always under review, as we learn more about MS, and more effective laboratory and clinical assessments are devised, neurological diagnosis of the condition generally requires at least two separately identifiable 'attacks' of symptoms, involving two different areas of the CNS. The diagnosis will also require relevant signs revealed during an examination by a neurologist, and will often be supported by laboratory tests. If you report only one 'attack', the neurologist may wish to wait until a second one occurs before making a formal diagnosis. The second 'attack' might not occur for a long time, indeed for several years. However, symptoms may be unclear, or it could be difficult to establish something as clear as an 'attack', or indeed there may be no remissions between attacks in some cases. In such a situation the diagnosis has to be mainly based on a concerted process of laboratory and clinical assessments: these can take some time in order to eliminate other possible causes for the symptoms.

I am seeing a neurologist soon. What will he do?

Three kinds of information are most commonly needed to help to establish a formal diagnosis of MS: your medical history, a neurological examination, and a series of tests (see the next section). The first and most important source of information in many ways is your *medical history*, obtained during a consultation with a doctor, usually a neurologist. This history focuses on the particular symptoms that you have experienced, the everyday activities affected by these symptoms, and the dates on which they first and subsequently occurred. Thus, keeping a diary of your own symptoms over time can be helpful for the doctor, although you will need to be aware that the doctor may be seeking special kinds of information that you may not have included in such a diary.

Usually a medical history will be accompanied by a second source of information, i.e. a *neurological examination*. The neurologist will try to establish, as objectively as possible, the extent to which your movements and reflexes (often called *functional abilities*) and some key sensory abilities (such as eyesight) are both different from those that would be expected in a person without MS, and are not typical of people with other medical conditions. This physical assessment, which may include a more general examination of your health, is not designed to reveal the cause of any symptoms immediately, but to discover the nature and degree of any problems and, as far as possible, help indicate the sites in the CNS that might be affected.

Tests

Can you tell me what tests I might be given in order to diagnose MS?

As discussed above, the third kind of information is gleaned from a range of tests; these may take place over a series of days, or even weeks. They often require special and expensive equipment or facilities that are used for other medical purposes as well.

- The most common tests given to people with suspected MS over the past few years have been what are described as evoked response tests. These tests are used to measure how quickly signals travel between the brain and most usually the ear (*auditory evoked response*) or the eye (*visually evoked response*). If the signal speed is lower than that which would be expected in a person without MS, then it indicates that there has been some damage to the nerve pathway along which the signal is conducted. Such damage may result from the demyelination associated with MS (see Chapter 1), or indeed may result from some other condition; thus the results are only indicative of the possibility of MS, they are not conclusive. Auditory evoked response measures the response to test signals heard by the ear; visual evoked response measures the response to test images seen by the eye. In both cases the tests are non-invasive – you just have small electrodes taped to your scalp to receive *electroencephalographic (EEG) recordings* on an external machine (Figure 4.1). You will only see or hear the test signals. Just to reassure you, in case you are worried about the electrodes, they have no electricity in them, they just measure the tiny electric currents that everyone has in their body.

- Another test that has been widely used in recent years is one which measures the characteristics of *cerebrospinal fluid* (CSF), a fluid which surrounds the brain and spinal cord. It has been found that many, although not all, people with MS have some differences in their CSF; this test could indicate that a diagnosis of the disease is a distinct possibility. In MS, the CSF may often have high levels of white blood cells and other indicators of inflammation – antibodies, myelin fragments and what is called *oligoclonal banding*: this indicates a problem in the immune system highly indicative of MS. For this test, a small quantity of spinal fluid is usually taken for laboratory analysis from the lower back area by what is called a *lumbar puncture* (or *spinal tap*). A lumbar puncture is an intrusive and uncomfortable process and, for this reason and because the test is not definitive (especially in the early stages of MS), neurologists are increasingly looking to use other less intrusive measures.

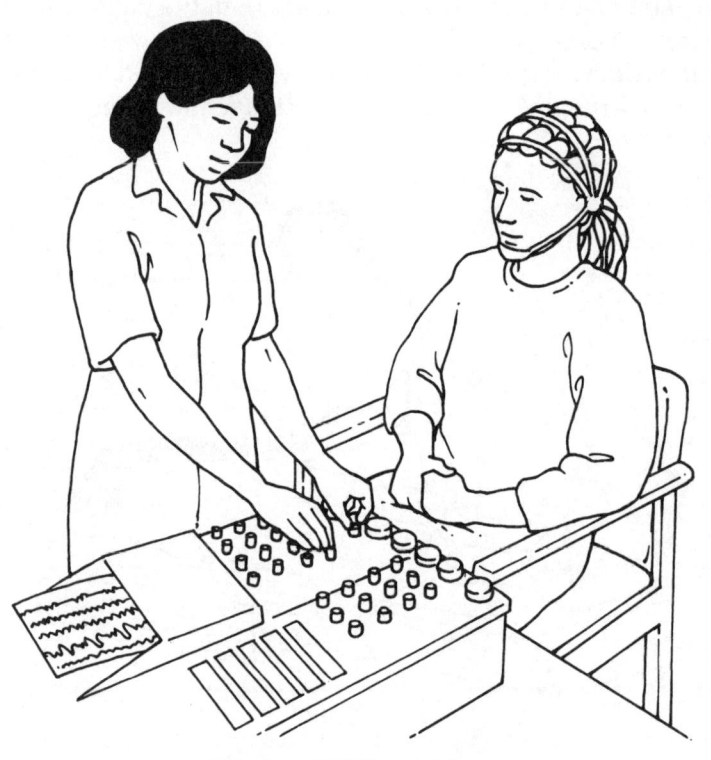

Figure 4.1 EEG procedure.

- The recent development of what are known as 'imaging' techniques has proved to be very important in providing additional and very detailed pictures of the process of demyelination inside the CNS. Earlier X-ray based techniques, such as the CT or CAT (*computerized axial tomography*) scan, still in use in some centres, can provide images of MS lesions, where demyelination has occurred or is occurring inside the CNS. However, the CAT scan shows these images with less detail (less resolution) and there is rather more (but still a very low) risk with these X-rays than with the newer imaging techniques.

- These new techniques, most of which centre on what is called *magnetic resonance imaging* (MRI), offer greatly increased resolution in images of any MS lesions present, and can be used much more freely and regularly than the older X-ray techniques, for they are based on the use of powerful magnets rather than X-rays. For MRI scans, you lie still on a table which moves through a 'tunnel' in the MRI machine (Figure 4.2); this

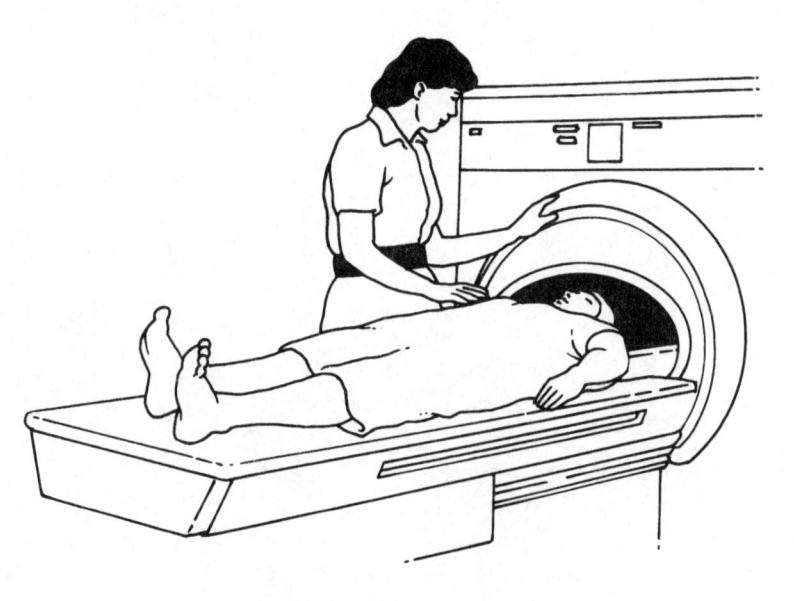

Figure 4.2 MRI scan procedure.

then sends images of what are, in effect, scans of 'slices' of your brain or spinal cord to a computer. These pictures are remarkably clear, and can provide a great deal of information about the activity of MS in these areas, especially if several images are taken over a period of time. However, MRI machines are very expensive, and the newer versions even more so, and thus not everyone with MS will have access to them. Perhaps even more significantly, an MRI scan is indicative rather than infallible, for early on in the disease a scan may not always be positive, even if the disease subsequently proves to be present. Lesions also arise from time to time as a normal process in all people, and increase in number naturally in older people. They are not necessarily a permanent feature of the brain or spinal cord – individual lesions may come and go, or change in size from one MRI scan to another. Furthermore, there is never an absolute correspondence between symptoms and what the lesion looks like. There may be both 'silent lesions', which are not related to any obvious symptom, and symptoms unrelated to the visible lesions. Thus whilst widespread or severe plaques (see Chapter 1) may be indicative of MS when consistently observed in follow-up scans, very careful clinical interpretation is always required.

In summary, the diagnosis of MS is still undertaken through your medical history, clinical and neurological assessment and judgement by a neurologist, despite the rapid scientific acceptance of the value of MRI scanning techniques. However, for research purposes, MRI scans in particular are proving enormously helpful in the documentation of changes inside the brain and spinal cord.

Receiving the news

Communicating any diagnosis that might affect a person's life is never easy. There is more about relationships between you and the health care team to be found in Chapter 16.

My doctor says that I 'probably' have MS. What does that mean and why the lack of certainty?

This is one of a trio of diagnostic categories that have been used a great deal by doctors investigating symptoms of MS, but are now used rather less, i.e. 'possible', 'probable' and 'definite' MS. The use of these terms has often coincided with the process of diagnosis. Early on in the diagnostic process, a doctor might conclude that MS was a 'possible' diagnosis amongst many other possible diagnoses which could account for the symptoms. Later, a doctor might conclude that MS was a 'probable' diagnosis, i.e. MS was the most likely explanation of the presenting symptoms. However, further tests, examinations or investigations were required to conclude that 'definite' MS existed, i.e. it was the only explanation for the symptoms. Traditionally time has been the key factor in distinguishing 'possible' from 'probable' and 'definite' MS, with the appearance of further 'relapses' and 'remissions' giving the doctor more grounds for deciding that the diagnosis was 'definite'. Many doctors have not been willing in the past to tell people that they have 'possible' or 'probable' MS, preferring to wait until they felt that MS was 'definite', although the former terms might appear on medical records. Now, with increasing medical openness, more people are being informed directly about 'possible' or 'probable' diagnoses.

I believe that my neurologist knew that I had MS several months before he actually told me. Why did he not tell me when he knew?

It is helpful at this point to distinguish between when a **definite diagnosis is made** by a doctor – which may take a long time – and **when it is told** to a person. In the latter case there may be additional reasons why people are not told their diagnosis, even if it has been (virtually) clinically made. The first is that the diagnosis is still provisional, i.e. the MS is still only a 'possible' or 'probable' diagnosis. Many doctors do not like giving information to someone that could significantly affect their future, when the diagnosis of MS is still – even a little – uncertain. They would prefer to wait until the diagnosis is absolutely definite. Secondly, a doctor may feel that the person diagnosed with MS is not in the best frame of mind to have the diagnosis communicated now – in other words, the doctor may feel that the person might be emotionally or otherwise seriously damaged by being told at this point. Therefore, on these clinical grounds, a doctor might delay telling someone for some weeks, or months, or occasionally for some years. With the arrival of the Patient's Charter, and a view that, ethically, it is the patient's 'right to know', the withholding of diagnoses on the very broad grounds of emotional or other harm to the person, or for other reasons, is now less common. Nevertheless, giving such a diagnosis is not easy for a doctor, and being told is not easy for the person with MS or the family. Thus it is a difficult time for everyone.

In the light of all these points, it is important that you let the doctor know clearly and directly if you wish to know your diagnosis as early as possible, whatever it may be – and even if at that time it is not yet a definite diagnosis of MS.

My neurologist gave the diagnosis of my MS to my wife first; I only learnt of it when she told me – almost by mistake – when we had a row about six months afterwards. I was very upset. Shouldn't I have been told first myself?

Research has shown that some neurologists were giving the diagnosis of MS first to the partner of the person with MS, although this is becoming increasingly uncommon now. It appeared that they thought that the 'healthy' person in the relationship would be better able to cope with the diagnosis, than the person 'ill' with MS. In fact, although this alleviated the doctor from a possibly difficult consultation with the person with MS, it placed a considerable burden on the partners; they may also have been told to decide for themselves when to tell the person with MS. In practice this kind of burden was a double problem: not only did they have to decide when to tell their partner, but they were also the privileged recipients of information which the partner did not have, leading to a lack of trust between them. Although most clinical practice has changed, and telling a partner first was in any case an ethically very dubious practice, it indicates the importance of greater openness in communicating an early diagnosis to the person with the disease.

I learnt my diagnosis from my case notes, which I happened to see when the physio came to see me in hospital. This was a shock. Why couldn't I have been told properly?

A significant minority of people with MS have learnt their diagnosis by chance. This happens surprisingly easily. It may be that the diagnosis had not been clinically definite and thus not been given to you formally by the doctor. He or she might have put a query about MS in your notes as a provisional diagnosis pending further confirmation. The doctor may have been waiting for an opportune time to communicate the diagnosis to you but had not yet done so. However, you do point to the fact that many professional staff may have access to your medical notes – legitimately – and there are many opportunities, often fortuitous, for you to (over)hear about them, or to see them. Physiotherapists, for example, may not know whether you have been told your diagnosis, and they may have unwittingly mentioned it to you. This issue suggests again that a communication of the diagnosis as early as possible, personally by the neurologist, is important.

As I would have wished, my neurologist told me bluntly and clearly that I had MS, but he didn't offer any hope for the future at all. I had to find out myself what I could do for the MS. Is this usually the case?

Although things are changing, many doctors have been concerned about giving too much 'hope' in relation to a disease like MS. They felt that giving hope was almost equivalent to indicating that the disease could be cured, which is unfortunately not yet so with MS. They also often felt that it was important, as the disease course could not be significantly altered, for the person with MS to live a life as fully as possible day by day, and knowing all the details of the diagnosis would not help in this process; thus detailed information about a pessimistic future (as they saw it) did not seem to be relevant in communicating the diagnosis.

However, most neurologists are now aware of the sensitivity needed to communicate the diagnosis of MS. Many more are offering what people with the disease feel they most require at this difficult point – what we might call sensitive frankness, but also continuing hope and support. There are a number of ways that can assist in ensuring a more positive relationship with a neurologist, beyond the point of diagnosis. Repeat visits are increasingly being offered so that people may raise additional queries that they may have been unable or unwilling to raise earlier when they were first diagnosed. Nurses or other health care team members who can be contacted readily about future concerns may also be introduced at that first communication. Booklets or addresses of organizations such as the MS Society (see Appendix 1 and 2) may be given to provide additional information. Thus the days of the blunt, but what we might call uninformative communication of the diagnosis (at least from the patient's point of view), are gradually disappearing. The best advice to someone who feels that they do not have the support that they would like is to seek a further meeting with the diagnosing neurologist or, if that fails, to contact the helpline of the MS Society for further information (see Appendix 1).

To my surprise, when my neurologist gave me my diagnosis at the hospital several people 'sat in' on it. I thought it should have been just my husband and myself and the neurologist. Why was that?

Managing MS is increasingly being seen as a professional team effort, in which specialist nurses, physiotherapists and other staff are fully involved. Although the neurologist continues to be the central figure, there is a move in many major MS hospitals to involve one or more other professional staff right from the beginning. The idea is to provide you with someone else who can assist you right from the start, in addition to the neurologist. However, on occasions, it may seem that there are too many people involved; sometimes trainee medical staff may be there, at this very sensitive time. If this is a problem for you, ask to see the neurologist alone.

5
Medical management of MS

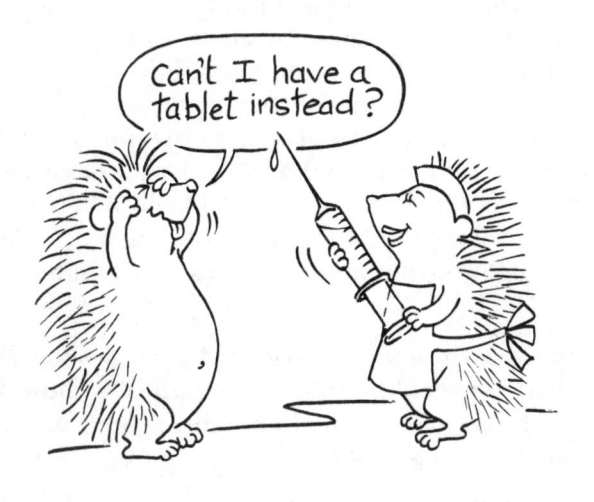

Despite claims that are made from time to time (see question in Chapter 5), at present there is no scientifically validated cure for MS. Neither can we prevent its onset, even though we now know, for example, that first-degree blood relatives of someone with MS, such as children and siblings (brothers and sisters), are at enhanced risk of the disease. This chapter discusses the issues of cure versus treatment, what medical therapies there are at present, and rehabilitation.

Cure versus treatment

One of the reasons why MS is such a difficult disease to cure is that, once the central nervous system (CNS) has been damaged, it involves a major repair process. It is not just a question of killing bacteria or stopping an infection – as in food poisoning or influenza – and then letting the body return, as it usually does, to its pre-existing state. In MS, there is continuing and often severe structural damage. Both the process of damage has to be prevented and the previous structural damage has to be repaired. Even if the destructive and demyelinating process in MS were halted (see Chapter 1), the existing damage, symptoms and consequences would still remain. This is why there is considerable interest at present in experimental work on drugs which may be able to 'remyelinate' damaged nerves. However, whether such remyelination – even if it were possible – would also lead to someone regaining pre-MS control of senses and muscles is open to question.

Most claims for a cure for MS have been made on the basis that the symptoms seem to have disappeared, temporarily at least. The claims are not usually based on a study of repair to the structural damage of MS in the body. Scientists would need to be convinced of this repair before considering that an individual's MS was 'cured'. The problem is that symptoms of MS can be dormant for very many years, and dramatic remissions in symptoms can also occur, but the damage to the CNS has not necessarily been repaired. Symptoms can always reappear, and there is a significant possibility that they will do so. Of course, you may say, 'Well, I don't give a damn as long as my symptoms go away – that's the same as a cure to me.' To a scientist, without other people with MS having exactly the same outcome by doing or taking the same thing, and without evidence that the underlying demyelination has been repaired, the disappearance of symptoms appears to be a temporary, although happy, coincidence.

Despite these difficulties, a lot of time, resources and research have been invested in finding a cure for MS. Everyone hopes that real progress can be made very soon.

How is treating MS different from curing it?

This is an important question, and often leads to misunderstand-
ings. You may think that 'treating' MS is tantamount to curing it.
However, when doctors or other health care workers talk about
'treating' MS, they do not mean 'curing' it. What they usually
mean is that there is some means of dealing with MS, or aspects
of it, through:

- ameliorating a symptom or its effects;

- preventing or lessening the degree or length of time of a
  'relapse';

- encouraging the early arrival of a 'remission';

- changing various aspects of your lifestyle that will make life
  with MS easier to manage.

**If MS is not curable now, what does medical treatment
achieve?**

In the absence of a cure, there are two basic approaches to treating MS medically.

There are several drugs that aim to suppress, minimize or halt
the destructive immune response, the inflammation and the
accompanying symptoms that occur when MS is in an active
phase, i.e. when a 'relapse' or 'attack' is occurring. Therapy
includes steroid-based drugs but they have little effect on the
underlying course of the disease. More recently, drugs based on
beta-interferon have been licensed for use in people with specific
relapsing-remitting forms of the disease, but they are now offering significantly more hope regarding the disease course itself.
There are also as many as 50 promising individual therapies
undergoing clinical trials at any one time, although few will end
up being used in clinical practice. Even if the drugs are successfully tested, it is unlikely that everyone with MS will benefit
substantially, for the drugs are often targeted to very specific
types of the disease.

The second basic approach is to assess and treat the individual symptoms (e.g. spasticity, continence difficulties, pain or fatigue) that result from the damage to the CNS. In this respect there is no single drug treatment – an 'MS drug' – for all the symptoms of MS because of the immense variation and different rates of progression in each individual. Also, as yet, no drug therapy is used exclusively for the treatment of symptoms of MS: most are aimed at specific symptoms which may be 'shared' with other medical conditions. Fortunately, MS is a condition where many symptoms can, in most cases, be relatively well managed for long periods of time.

Beta-interferon

Lots of people I know are now talking about beta-interferons, as an exciting and effective new way of controlling MS. It sounds almost like a cure to me. Is it?

No. Beta-interferons are not a cure for MS. However, we think it is fair to say that they are one of the biggest advances in MS over the past few years.

Interferons are naturally occurring substances in the body, produced in response to 'invasion' by a foreign substance, such as a virus. The problem has been to isolate, synthesize and test the various types of interferons, and to evaluate their effectiveness in MS. Now after years of scientific work, two different kinds of beta-interferons have shown a significant effect in MS by reducing the number and severity of its 'attacks': beta-interferon 1b (trade name Betaferon) and, more recently, beta interferon 1a (trade names Avonex and Rebif). They seem to stabilize the immune system and, in the case of beta-interferon 1a, there is increasing evidence that it may also slow disease progression. A newer drug is similarly effective: copolymer 1 (trade name Copaxone), but this is not a beta-interferon. There are a number of other promising drugs, not just based on beta-interferons, currently in the clinical trial stage. Results from a number of these trials are expected over the next few months, and the trial results may prove important (see Chapter 17).

These beta-interferon drugs sound almost too good to be true. Can they help everyone with MS?

The answer is that it is not clear at present. The drugs were first tested on people with specific kinds of relapsing-remitting MS, mainly those in the earlier stages of MS and who could walk (in the jargon, those who were *ambulant*). This was because it was easier to demonstrate the effectiveness of the drugs on people who were more mildly affected and who were having relatively regular 'relapses'. Findings of several trials showed that these people had a (statistically) significantly lower rate of relapses compared to a group of others who did not take the drugs and, furthermore, when they did have a relapse, it was likely to be less severe.

Now we have to be careful here. This did not mean that **everyone** who took the drugs had a lower rate of, or less severe, relapses, than the other group, only that **(statistically) more** did. In other words, there were still some people who took the drugs who did not benefit a great deal from them. We must also remember that the criteria for 'relapsing-remitting MS' in the trials were drawn very tightly; many people have types of MS that are not covered by the first trial findings. New trials are underway to test whether these other people might benefit as well. However, because it is more difficult to test the effects of such drugs in people with more complicated relapsing-remitting, or progressive types of MS, the findings are taking some time, although initial results are promising. Beta-interferons may have less effect on people whose disease progression is very substantial. As a result the drugs are currently *licensed* for use only in those people with MS who fit the original clinical trial criteria.

What do you mean by a licensed drug?

Although the findings of clinical trials on particular drugs may be promising, or even striking, in many countries – including Britain and the United States – there are formal government-supported organizations which make the final decision as to whether doctors may use a drug in their clinical practice and, if so, for which groups of patients and under what conditions. In the United States, this Agency is the FDA (Food and Drug Agency); in Britain, the Committee on the Safety of Medicines. These Agencies are also responsible for monitoring the side effects of drugs through reports from doctors on how their patients have reacted to the drugs. The Agencies may sometimes withdraw a drug – for example, if its side effects become unacceptable – or they may vary the types of patients to which, or types of conditions under which, the drug can be administered.

It is important to make another point: the licensing of a drug does not necessarily mean that it will be used. Further decisions will be made by governments, by health trusts and authorities, and by individual doctors, on financial as well as other grounds. In the case of very expensive drugs, such as the beta-interferons, financial aspects might be critical for deciding whether the drugs are made available, despite evidence of their clinical effectiveness. The Government in Britain has recently set up a body called *NICE* (National Institute for Clinical Excellence) to review the scientific and clinical evidence for new drugs and other healthcare interventions, in order to judge their effectiveness in relation to their cost. The Government has also indicated that unless NICE has approved a particular drug or intervention, it will not be offered through the National Health Service. The beta-interferons will probably be one of the first sets of drugs to be assessed by NICE.

How do you take beta-interferon? I've heard that you need injections, and I hate jabs!

Beta-interferons may be administered in different ways. The first beta-interferon (1b – trade name Betaferon) to be approved is administered by injection *subcutaneously* (just below the skin) every other day. The second beta-interferon to be approved (1a – trade name Avonex) is administered by injection *intramuscularly* (directly into the muscles) every week. The third beta-interferon to be approved (1a – trade name Rebif) is also administered subcutaneously three times a week. The different mode of administration is based on what has proved in clinical trials to be the best way of ensuring the effectiveness of the drug. Subcutaneous injections have been given in the past by a doctor or a nurse, not only to check that it is given correctly, but to monitor whether it is given at all – people are sometimes forgetful about administering any drug. However, this is a time-consuming and expensive process and, following experience in the United States, there are now moves to let people self-administer the drug, rather like the insulin with which people with diabetes inject themselves. As far as a second beta-interferon (1a – Avonex) is concerned, intramuscular injections have to be undertaken by a doctor (or nurse). None of the drugs can at present be taken orally; they are proteins and likely to be broken down by the digestive processes, making them less effective, or possibly even ineffective. However, a range of developments and trials is taking place to test whether other methods of administration are better and more effective.

What about the side effects of beta-interferon? Don't all powerful drugs have side effects?

One of the problems of the very early trials with the beta-interferons was the wide range of side effects, largely restricted now to two sets of symptoms experienced with beta-interferon 1b (Betaferon). The first set relates to what can be best described as 'flu-like symptoms that many, perhaps most, people experience in the first few months of treatment. These are generally mild and can be managed with ordinary analgesics (pain relievers), and they disappear in almost everyone after those first few months. The second set relates to problems at the injection site – often blotches or some pain may occur – that most people experienced initially and about half some years later. Such reactions are more of an irritation than anything else. Occasionally more serious reactions have been reported – in a few cases serious enough to warrant stopping treatment – but this has been a very rare occurrence.

As far as beta-interferon 1a drugs (Avonex and Rebif) are concerned, similar types of side effects were experienced, but at a lower rate.

We should just note, however, that the use of beta-interferons for MS is relatively new, and so we do not know at present if there are any longer term side effects about which we should be concerned. This is, of course, a particular issue in MS where people usually live with MS through several decades.

I recently heard about beta-interferon and how it could help MS, so I went to my GP to ask for it. She said she could not prescribe it. Why?

It has been decided that, because the beta-interferon based drugs are so new, only specific types of MS are to be targeted; side effects require careful monitoring and can be prescribed only by specialists, i.e. neurologists. Thus, all your GP can do is to refer you to a neurologist, based in a hospital, for assessment, with a view to the possible use of beta-interferons.

Steroids

You have talked a lot about these new beta-interferon drugs, but my friend has been given steroid drugs when she had an attack of MS. What are these?

The use of steroid-based drugs for 'attacks' or 'relapses' of MS has been the standard treatment for MS for some years, and many people may still find that this is the first line of treatment offered to them.

There are several types of steroid drugs. The two that mainly used are:

- *adrenocorticosteroids* (such as ACTH – AdrenoCorticoTrophic Hormone), the most commonly used steroid in MS; and

- *glucocorticosteroids* (such as prednisolone, given by mouth; or methylprednisolone, usually given through a drip, intra-venously).

There is substantial evidence that both types reduce the inflammation at active disease sites in the CNS and, in particular, reverse disruptions of the blood–brain barrier (BBB) (see Chapter 3) that may occur when the disease is active. These effects, in turn, should reduce the duration and degree of symptoms. However, most studies suggest that the effects of steroids are relatively short term, perhaps lasting a few weeks, although there have been one or two studies which suggest tantalizingly that there may be far longer positive effects of the combined short-term use of methylprednisolone and prednisolone.

By and large, ACTH in practice is gradually being replaced by the use of methylprednisolone and prednisolone, but there is widespread debate amongst neurologists about the most appropriate steroid and mode of administration in MS. People with MS are likely to come across different ways in which steroids are currently given – intravenously administered methylprednisolone (called IVMP for short) normally requires a hospital stay for one to several days, depending on precisely how the drug is administered. There may need to be other hospital stays for assessment purposes.

Overall there is a sense, at the moment, that further definitive trials to assess the most effective particular steroid, dose and mode of administration in MS, are now almost a waste of time and resources, as newer drugs – such as the beta-interferons and others – show so much more promise for the control of MS, in relation not only to relapses, but also possibly to the progress of the disease.

I have progressive MS. My doctor says that neither beta-interferons nor steroids are going to help me. Is that really the case?

We must distinguish here between 'primary progressive' MS, where MS seems to get gradually but perceptibly worse right from the start without any significant remissions (or indeed relapses), and 'secondary progressive' MS, where the progression follows an earlier relapsing-remitting course. In the former case there is less compelling evidence at present that the current therapies, i.e. beta-interferons, steroids, or indeed the newer copolymer 1, substantially affect the longer term course of the disease, although there have been some very recent more hopeful findings in this respect. The focus of drug trials has been on evaluating effects in the relapsing-remitting form of the disease, for it is far easier to test efficacy in this form. In the case of secondary progression, as it is preceded by a relapsing-remitting phase, such people will probably benefit through some of the therapies, especially beta-interferon, which may have some effect on modifying the earlier phase of the disease. However, the results of some very recent trials have shown that the beta-interferons may slow down the course of the disease over a three- to four-year period. Nevertheless, at present, drug therapy for primary progressive MS is still mainly to manage any symptoms as they appear. However, given the evidence that beta-interferons can produce some benefits for both relapsing-remitting and secondary progressive MS, research is now increasingly interested in their potential effects in primary progressive MS.

Can I take both one of the new interferon drugs and steroids at the same time?

The answer is yes, but only after careful assessment by your neurologist. Even if you are taking either beta-interferon 1b or beta-interferon 1a, you may have a relapse, but probably to a lesser degree than you would have done without the treatment. In this situation, you may well be offered steroids – possibly a combination of methylprednisolone and prednisolone. The objective is to provide an additional means of reducing the inflammation, despite the use of beta-interferons, and reduce your symptoms.

It sounds from what you have said about the promise of the new drugs, that I hardly need to worry about other ways of managing my MS. Is that so?

Definitely not! Many people with MS for the foreseeable future will need professional support services and assistance at some time, to manage the changes in their lifestyles, and to monitor effects of any new drugs. Depending on the precise nature of your MS and its effects, such services may include nursing, physiotherapy, occupational therapy, speech therapy, psychological assessment and support, counselling and advice on housing, employment, financial and other similar issues (see later chapters). Such professional support services for all the many consequences of MS have not previously been adequate, in fact often woefully inadequate and ill-coordinated. Despite serious financial constraints, there are now many attempts underway locally to provide better coordinated services and support.

Where can I find out more about the drugs that my GP has prescribed for me, and the side effects that they may cause?

Although it can appear to be a little morbid focusing on the side effects of the drugs prescribed for you, this is a very important issue. By and large, if drugs have powerful effects on what they are intended to control, they also have powerful side (that is unwanted) effects on other things. By understanding the possible side effects of your drugs, you will not be taken by surprise if they occur, and will be able to tell your GP or neurologist about them, if they are worrying you.

Your medical practitioner (GP or neurologist) should discuss possible side effects with you when he or she is prescribing your drug(s), including any that can occur from a combination of two or more. If not, you should ask explicitly about them. If you are still unclear or concerned, the pharmacist where you get your prescriptions has expert knowledge about drugs and their effects, and should be willing to answer questions about them. Furthermore, they can inform you about over-the-counter drug therapies that you may buy, and their potential side effects and interactions with other drugs. Several organizations (including the Consumers' Association and British Medical Association) publish excellent family health guides which contain detailed and up-to-date information about drugs and other treatments. It is vital that you use a British edition of any guide, as brand names are frequently changed from country to country. Some titles are included in Appendix 2 at the back of this book.

Rehabilitation

I have been offered 'in-patient rehabilitation' in hospital. What will that mean?

'Rehabilitation' is perhaps the new watchword of longer term care in MS. Broadly it means professional care targeted to achieve your maximum potential. With the newer team approach, and a concern about making treatment as (cost) effective as possible, the use of in-patient care for this purpose has become a matter of considerable interest. Regional Rehabilitation Units have been created in recent years for the support of people with many conditions, but there are also other more specialist MS rehabilitation units or programmes. At present there are only a limited number of places available on these rehabilitation programmes, and there is a selection process involved, usually on the basis of who might be expected medically to get the most benefit.

6
Complementary therapies and MS

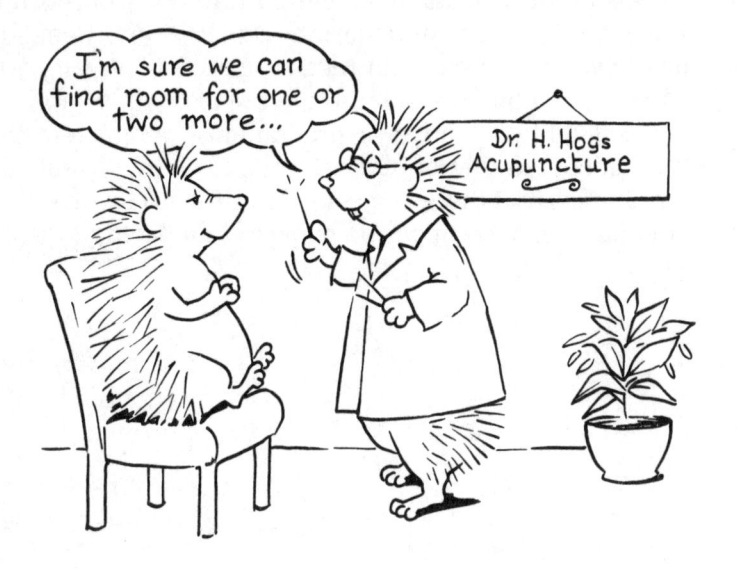

When there is no current scientifically accepted cure for a disease, other people – including people with MS – understandably want to find the cause, means of management or indeed cure for the disease. Many people over the last 30 or 40 years have claimed that they have the answer to MS. One problem, of course, is that because MS is so variable and unpredictable it is relatively easy to find something that coincides with it becoming either worse (a relapse), or better (a remission). The difficult problem is to find out whether there really is a connection.

A distinguishing characteristic of complementary therapies is their focus on the 'whole person', not just (or even at all) on particular symptoms, but on the use of the body's own healing powers to meet the challenge of diseases. Partly because of the broad focus of such therapies, their assumed effects on overall body systems, and their gearing to individuals as much as to diseases, they are very difficult to evaluate in formal scientific terms. Many have not yet been scientifically studied, although both their practitioners and their patients may have a very high opinion of their value. Complementary therapies are also very varied in nature and are often based on different (and competing) views of how the body – and mind – operates.

Where to go

How can I find a practitioner in a particular complementary therapy?

Finding a competent practitioner for a complementary therapy is not always easy. There is little statutory regulation for qualifications or practice for most of the therapies and therapists. However, the best ways of finding a practitioner are through:

- an MS resource or therapy centre, where often other people with MS and staff in the centre will have experience of particular therapists;

- a recommendation or referral from a neurologist, GP or other health care professional;

- registers set up by the professional bodies of whichever therapy you are interested in;

- referral for homeopathy to one of the NHS hospitals providing this service;

- contacting the British Complementary Medicine Association, or the Institute of Complementary Medicine (see Appendix 1).

Even if you are confident about the advice that you are given by others you trust, you ought to ask questions about how practitioners in the therapy are trained and licensed; whether they are insured for malpractice, negligence or accident; and how complaints are handled. One of the key things is to try and ensure that whichever therapist you go to has a good understanding of MS. Both of you should be able to evaluate its benefits.

There seem to be a lot of benefits from complementary medicine, and even my regular doctor has mentioned some of the methods available. Who will pay for complementary therapy if I choose to have any?

Complementary and alternative therapies range from the practical to the bizarre and the terms 'complementary' and 'alternative' disguise the tradition and respect that many forms of therapy outside the medical profession command. Many alternative therapies (acupuncture and osteopathy to name only two) are increasingly recognized as having significant benefits and can, in certain circumstances and limited geographic areas, be made available through the NHS. Many GPs are now more willing to accept and recommend alternatives. At present you will almost inevitably have to pay for your own treatment. The appropriate registration bodies can provide details of registered practitioners in your local area and provide guidance on how much you might expect to pay. You may find the addresses of these registration bodies through the British Complementary Medicine Association or the Institute of Complementary Medicine (see Appendix 1).

Complementary therapies

We discuss the role of evening primrose oil in Chapter 11. Here we consider some other substances that have been hitting the headlines.

There has been a lot of publicity recently about people with MS using cannabis to help reduce spasticity and pain. If it can help me, I should like to try it. How can I obtain it?

One of the major MS symptoms is spasticity, often associated with some pain. Conventional treatments for spasticity are dealt with in Chapter 8, but an increasing number of people are using cannabis. As with other complementary therapies, you have to balance benefits against costs, **but** there is one very important addition – cannabis is illegal in Britain, and cannot be prescribed.

However, there is evidence that an increasing number of people with MS are using cannabis on an occasional or sometimes regular basis; it has become a very difficult issue because, although they do feel that they gain from taking it, they are having to balance what they feel is a significant reduction in their symptoms against committing an illegal act. Using the drug in any form is illegal, including 'inactivated' tinctures with limited narcotic effects. Growing, buying, selling and using cannabis carry penalties of heavy fines and jail sentences, even when there is a medical justification for its use. There is a group campaigning for a change in the law (the Alliance for Cannabis Therapeutics) to allow the use of cannabis for medically designated purposes, and if you feel strongly about the issue you may wish to join this group (see Appendix 1).

Some small scale inconclusive research studies have shown that cannabis might be helpful in controlling spasticity, muscle spasms, tremor, pain and fatigue. Note that the active agents in cannabis are many and at present it is not known which are responsible for producing the effects of cannabis in MS. Pharmaceutical companies are now very interested in the potential effects of cannabis on symptoms of MS, and have synthesized some of the most likely and effective agents in the substance. There is currently a major clinical trial underway on cannabis and specific symptoms such as pain and spasticity (and others are planned), and it will be interesting to see how this trial develops in due course.

There have been many TV documentaries and newspaper stories written about revolutionary new therapies for MS. What do you think of them?

Yes, indeed there have! In general it is sensible to be very cautious about any new therapy. The variability of MS is notorious, as is the possibility of substantial spontaneous remissions, and so it is important to wait for the results of appropriate clinical trials. If there is a 'breakthrough', you are likely to hear about it very quickly from other sources, such as the MS Society. The main questions to ask yourself about new 'wonder' therapies are:

- What detailed evidence is there that the new therapy can help MS?

- Has the treatment been endorsed by the MS Society or other leading medical research centres on MS?

- What are the possible side effects?

- How expensive is it in relation to the assumed benefits?

- How easy is it to acquire?

- Are its practitioners well trained, professionally recognized and insured?

- Would it involve you giving up, or not taking conventional medical advice or treatments?

What are all these new therapies?

Here are some of the most recently mentioned ideas:

- A special combination of substances consisting of **tricyclic antidepressants**, a substance called phenylalanine, and subcutaneous (below the skin) injections of **vitamin B12** has been extensively written about. The therapy received very wide publicity and led to much controversy but, at the time of the publicity, it had not been tested in a formal clinical trial. This is now happening and in due course the results of the trial will become available.

- **Hyperbaric oxygen therapy** (HBO), which basically consists of breathing oxygen under high pressure, usually by sitting or lying in a large pressurized chamber, proved to be one of the more popular complementary therapies for MS in the 1980s and early 1990s. The former national charity Action for Research in Multiple Sclerosis was instrumental in supporting the installation and running of pressurized chambers in many local therapy centres. A substantial number of these chambers are still in operation in centres now run by Regional Federations of MS Therapy Centers. Although the main stream of scientific opinion is not in favour of this therapy, a considerable number of people with MS still use it in the Therapy Centres. Clinical trials showed that HBO did seem to reduce urinary symptoms (such as incontinence) and fatigue, but had no significant effect on other symptoms or the course of the disease.

- **Herbal medicine** has become popular in recent years, with practitioners operating with a range of different approaches. Although herbal remedies sound very benign and safe, they can be very powerful and can have side effects. It is important that any practitioner is very well trained in the properties, toxic as well as beneficial, of the herbs that they use, and also has a good knowledge of MS. Certain herbal remedies may help relieve some symptoms, but there is no evidence that it can alter the course of MS. Note also that some Chinese herbal remedies contain animal products.

- **Botulinum toxin** is an unconventional therapy designed to relieve muscle spasms, to improve control of muscles and to relieve the pain that can accompany spasticity. It is a very toxic substance in its original form, and has been specially prepared for therapeutic purposes. It has undergone more testing than other unconventional therapies, but with very variable results, and the therapy may need to be repeated to maintain its effects. As far as we are aware there is no centre giving this treatment for MS in Britain.

- **Bee and wasp stings and snake venoms** have received considerable publicity over the last few years. Most of their use has been unauthorized, unevaluated, untested and, moreover, undertaken outside the control of the regulatory authorities in Britain and Europe. A more positive longer term view is that many natural toxins are complex products and once these compounds have been identified, isolated and tested, one of them **might** prove to have some effect in MS.

Complementary treatments

Some of my friends with MS have told me to try various other complementary or alternative therapies to help me. Can you list some that are available?

There are many new and not so new practices that have been tried by people with MS. Overall the key issue is to get good information about the therapy, so that you can make an informed judgement about whether it will be of value to you.

- **Homeopathy** is a system of therapy in which minute doses of a substance are taken on the basis that these will cure or control symptoms that would be produced by the very same substance in much larger doses. Many scientists argue that the doses are so small that they cannot be detected using laboratory instruments and are thus sceptical about the efficacy of homeopathy, but homeopaths believe that their system of therapy is both effective and safe. Homeopaths normally focus on the person as much as the disease, and thus any specific symptoms of MS are only one aspect of the person's life and experiences, used to determine a relevant therapy. As might be expected from homeopathic theories, if a remedy is given which appears to be relevant to the symptom, an initial 'aggravation' of the symptom may occur – in other words, it can get worse – before any improvement is noted. It is difficult to undertake formal trials of the value of such therapy, although more are now being undertaken. Some have shown benefit for certain symptoms, but not yet in MS.

- **Acupuncture**, in its traditional form, is based on the idea that energy (*chi* or *qi*) flows round the body through channels (called *meridians*) which become blocked at times of illness and stress. Acupuncturists use the insertion of very fine needles at key points on these meridians, unblocking energy flows to help restore health. Acupressure (often known as *shiatzu*) works on a similar principle, but uses pressure from fingers or thumbs at these energy points. Results of some scientific studies suggest that in certain circumstances acupuncture does appear to relieve pain (although acupuncturists claim more general benefits), but it would be wise to seek a diagnosis of any source of pain that you have from your GP or neurologist, before undertaking such a treatment, in case there are other causes that need to be treated.

- **Yoga** is widely used by many people with MS, and there are now both specialist centres and teachers for them. From a practical point of view, in many respects yoga can be seen as providing a form of exercise which is known to be helpful in keeping your muscles working, as well as a way of calming of the mind, helpful in countering depression, stress and fatigue. One advantage may be that, in addition to its emphasis on slow movement, and peace and calm, once you have received some training, you can undertake the exercises at home. Its emphasis on deep and controlled breathing can also be helpful, particularly if your posture is not what it should be, or if you are sitting for long periods. The main concern with yoga and MS is that you should work well within your limitations in a relaxed way, and be careful not to push yourself too far, or raise your body temperature, as this may increase fatigue. If you are undergoing, or have been undergoing physiotherapy, it may be an idea to consult your physiotherapist about starting yoga. You can obtain more information about yoga from the Yoga for Health Foundation which runs special classes for people with MS and other conditions, or from the Royal

London Homeopathic Trust (Yoga Therapy Centre) (see Appendix 1).

- **Aromatherapy** is usually a massage with specific oils. The oils used are called 'essential oils'; they are very concentrated, and should always be used in a carrier oil during massage. They must not be taken by mouth. Some of the oils should not be used if you are pregnant, or have certain other conditions, such as epilepsy, and it is crucial that you let your aromatherapist know about these. The relaxing and gentle forms of massage are potentially of considerable value, not only in relaxing muscles and reducing spasticity, but also in promoting a general sense of well-being. It is very important that you check what form of massage the therapist is offering, and ensure that the therapist has been well trained and, above all, knows about MS, because some forms of massage are very vigorous and seek to realign the musculature of the body that such therapists believe is out of alignment in many, if not most, people. These realigning forms of massage should be avoided by people with MS. However, most aromatherapists use gentler forms of massage.

- **Reflexology** is a therapy based on the idea that energy and other flows in the body are linked to, indeed terminate, at key points in the feet, providing a 'map' of key organs and systems in the body. It is believed that problems in all areas of the body can thus be identified and indeed treated through manipulating the feet. Some people with MS have indicated that they have found this therapy helpful and relaxing, although there is no formal evidence that it affects the course of MS, or even major symptoms of the disease. However, as a relaxing therapy, it may benefit some people with the condition.

- **Chiropractic** is a long-standing approach to health founded on a particular view of the ways in which the human body works and may be managed. Practitioners manipulate the bones, muscles and tissues, especially around the spine, to enhance health. In chiropractic, the focus is mainly the nervous system, enhancing the blood supply around key tissues. Practitioners can use a variety of techniques which vary in strength. A course of treatment is usually composed of short sessions spaced out over several months. It recommends itself particularly for back pain and persistent headaches. In very rare instances, manipulation of the spinal column can cause lasting damage, so always ensure that you consult a qualified chiropractor and that you discuss your MS fully before any treatment begins.

- **Osteopathy** is a relatively long-standing, well regulated and trained profession compared to other complementary therapies, and a practitioner must be registered with the General Osteopathic Council (see Appendix 1). Like chiropractic, practitioners manipulate the bones, muscles and tissues, especially around the spine, to enhance health, particularly through working with the skeletal structure, bones and joints. Treatment may involve established medical diagnostic procedures (including X-rays and standard biochemical tests) in addition to manipulation of joints, rhythmic exercise and stretching. Osteopathy can improve mobility in some affected joints. Cranial osteopathy involves gentle manipulation of the bones of the head and spine.

7
Problems with urination and bowels

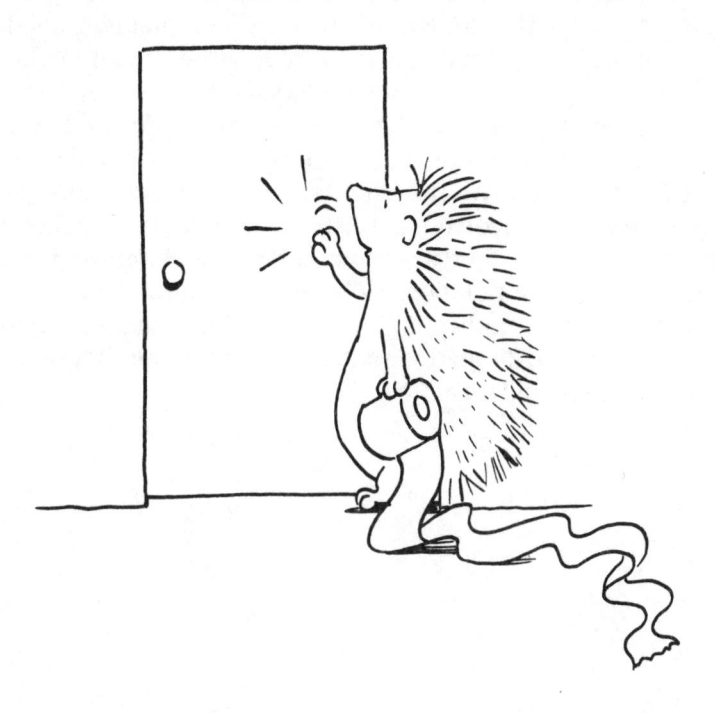

Urinary and bowel function problems probably cause the most inconvenience to a person with MS. They can be embarrassing to cope with and may be the ones most difficult to discuss with your doctor.

Managing urination problems

I am very embarrassed about wetting myself on occasions and losing control of my bladder. Is this the result of my MS?

Almost certainly it is. Problems with control of your bladder is one of the most difficult issues to deal with in MS, despite being a very common symptom. Only very recently has this difficult personal and social problem been discussed as openly as it should have been; increasing expertise and resources are now being devoted to dealing with it.

It is worth explaining some of the basic problems that may arise. Urinary control is very closely linked to particular nerves in the spinal cord, and if these are damaged by MS, as they often are, then urinary control will be affected. Normally the bladder fills gradually, and then signals are sent via the spinal cord to the brain that you should urinate; once you are in a position to urinate (e.g. on a toilet), signals are sent back to contract some muscles and relax others to release the urine. In MS this flow of signals backwards and forwards to and from the brain can be interrupted, distorted or destroyed.

There are several kinds of urinary control which might then be affected:

- People may wish to urinate more often than before (a problem of *frequency*). When people have frequency at night, i.e. needing to urinate several times during the night, it is called *nocturia*.

- They may wish to urinate immediately (a problem of *urgency*).

- They may find it difficult to begin to, or to continue to urinate (a problem of *hesitancy*).

- They may fail to empty their bladder (a problem of *voiding*).

- They may urinate involuntarily – either just dribbling a little, or sometimes even more (a problem of *incontinence*).

A number of these problems may occur at the same time, with the nervous system failing to coordinate the necessary muscles. Thus, for example, it is possible to have both urgency and hesitancy at the same time, where there is an urgent need to urinate but you still cannot easily do so, and this can, in some people, also be linked to dribbling (incontinence).

Most people with MS have one or more of these problems, either on a temporary or continuing basis. In general the more serious the MS, the more serious your urinary symptoms are likely to be. Early in the disease any problems will probably concern either or both frequency and urgency.

Some people with MS, who have had problems with frequency, have been taught pelvic floor exercises that have helped to tone the muscles in and around the urinary system. This is sometimes called 'bladder squeezing' and it has helped to decrease the frequency problems in some people. As a general rule, exercising your pelvic floor muscles is a good idea, although other help may well be required to help your urinary problems, as many of them are not easily controlled by such exercises, especially as the MS becomes more severe.

I often have to go to 'the loo' very urgently. Is there anything I can do to control this? It is very embarrassing.

The issue of urinary *urgency*, often combined with wanting to urinate more frequently is one of the most difficult problems for people with MS, earlier in the disease. It is usually caused by the bladder not storing the urine properly, or a lack of coordination between the storage and emptying process. Mainly it is wise to plan ahead whenever you leave home, and ensure that there are always toilet facilities within easy reach, but there are other aids. *Anticholinergic drugs* can help substantially. The most widely used is oxybutin chloride (Ditropan) which, in effect, blocks the nerve signals that trigger the muscles to release urine. This can be very effective, but is also associated with side effects, such as a dry mouth, because the drug blocks the nerve signals to the salivary glands as well. Indeed, without a dry mouth, it may be that the dose of the drug is too low. Unfortunately, it may also increase the likelihood of constipation, and at very high doses there may be problems with your sight. Often you have to experiment under the guidance of your doctor to find the most appropriate dose level controlling urgency with minimal other side effects. Another anticholinergic drug, propantheline, can be used, although trials have shown it to be slightly less effective than oxybutin. An antidepressant such as imipramine (Tofranil) may also be prescribed – not for depression, but because it has been found to have a similar effect in controlling urgency.

You may not need to take one of these drugs continuously, but you could use it for a particularly important event or journey when you need to avoid urinating for some time. For peace of mind on particular occasions, you could use a protective pad to absorb urine, in case you have 'an accident'. As a final point, people who have urinary problems often also have mobility problems – the nerves controlling both legs and the urinary system are situated close together – so the difficulties experienced through frequency and urgency are often compounded.

Because I have so many problems with urination, I have now decided to drink as little as I can. It seems to help. Is this a good way of controlling my problems?

Definitely no. Indeed this can be quite dangerous. Many people with MS have problems not only with urgency or frequency, but also with some urine retention in the bladder. If this is the case, reducing fluid intake substantially increases the risk of urinary infection, because urine as a waste product is not being diluted. A useful rule of thumb is the colour of your urine: if it is dark yellow to brown in colour then almost certainly you are not taking in enough fluid.

There are some useful guidelines which should help you:

• Drink at least 2 litres (or just over 3 pints) of liquid a day.

• In general, an acid urine helps keep infections at bay.

• Decrease your intake of citrus juices.

- Foods and substances which neutralize acidity, including antacid preparations such as sodium bicarbonate, should be eaten less often, as should dried vegetables.

- Increase your intake of proteins.

- Drink cranberry juice, and eat plums and prunes regularly. Cranberry juice will also help to provide the vitamin C lost through reducing the intake of citrus fruits.

I have two sorts of difficult problems with urination. One is that I can't easily start urinating, even though I want to go, and the other is that I still have a feeling that my bladder is relatively full, even after I have been. Can I do anything about these problems?

Both are frustrating problems. As far as the hesitancy goes – not being able to start urinating – you might adopt one of a number of approaches. Often urination starts after a couple of minutes, so be patient! Sometimes tapping very lightly on your lower abdomen – but not too hard – will help; this often produces a reflex reaction of urination. There have recently been trials of a hand-held vibrating device which, when held against your lower abdomen if you are still sensitive in this area, seems to work quite well by increasing urinary flow and leaving less urine in your bladder. However, the bladder is rarely completely emptied in this way, and the technique is probably most useful for people with relatively mild MS. Of course, other time-honoured techniques may work, including turning a tap on and hearing the sound of running water! A more direct method is to stimulate the urethra gently, at the tip of the penis or just above the vagina, with a clean finger or damp tissue.

If you have the feeling that your bladder is still full, this may need further investigation. It is important that your bladder is as empty as possible after you have urinated, not least to try and avoid an infection. Intermittent self-catheterization (ISC) may help, as may anticholinergic drugs. If you need further advice, make an appointment to see your doctor or, if possible, your neurologist.

Will my urinary problems ever get better?

The symptoms of MS are unpredictable, and thus no single pattern emerges. Remissions may be associated with your symptoms getting better for a period of time, and on a day-to-day basis the symptoms can fluctuate with 'good days' and 'bad days'. However, it would be unwise to hope for a significant and long-term improvement in urinary problems, unless new therapies are found that can repair both the relevant nerve demyelination and the associated loss of function.

Managing bowel function

I always seem to be constipated. Is this a symptom of the MS, or something else?

Even for people without MS constipation is a very common problem, as evidenced by the number of remedies available in chemist shops, but there are some special issues that may make constipation worse, more frequent, more continuous or, indeed, more problematic for people with MS.

It is not as easy to explain bowel problems, especially constipation, being caused by MS as urinary symptoms. A range of different and intrinsically separate processes together control or support bowel function. Some people with MS, whose spinal cord is particularly affected and who have significant bladder problems, have no major bowel dysfunction; others, who have few other serious MS signs and symptoms, seem to have major bowel dysfunction, and particularly constipation. Thus, some doctors have suggested that bowel dysfunction is rather like fatigue (see Chapter 9) in the sense of having no clear and obvious neurological cause. However, when MS becomes more severe, it is much more likely that people with the disease will have difficulty evacuating their bowels, as various body systems linked to this process become less efficient. You may need to undergo detailed medical investigation and get help for this problem.

For most people with MS who have constipation, especially in the earlier stages of the disease, the advice is very similar to that for other people with the same problem. In particular:

- Your diet should be high in fibre (e.g. bran, cereals, fruit and vegetables), which allows stools to pass more easily through the intestinal tract.

- Fluid intake should also be increased for the same reason.

- Getting as much exercise as possible can help, although clearly this particular advice will be less easy to follow by those who are bed-bound or using wheelchairs. In this latter case seek advice from your physiotherapist.

- Proprietary bulking agents (such as Fibogel, Metamucil, Mucasil), and stool softeners, can help produce regular motions.

- You could use laxatives, suppositories or enemas occasionally if all else fails, but be careful about using any of these too regularly, because they can actually increase constipation if overused, by slowing down natural bowel function still further.

- Finally, make time for regular daily bowel habits (see below).

I know all about the problems that people with MS have with their bladder – I have some myself – but I have recently been having some bowel problems. Do people with MS get 'bowel incontinence' like some get 'urinary incontinence'?

This has been a neglected area in MS. Recent research has revealed that something like two-thirds of people with MS have some bowel problems and, over several months, nearly half, in one study, had some degree of what is described as *faecal* or *bowel incontinence*. Of course, what appears to be an involuntary release of faeces produces a very unpleasant situation. Occasionally, there may be a link between urinary and bowel incontinence (from weakened muscles, from spasms in the intestinal area induced by MS, or from a full bowel pressing on the bladder), but the link is not always definite.

The exact causes of bowel incontinence are not always easy to find, even in the few centres with special facilities for investigating these issues, but there are several pointers to what may be happening in many cases. Involuntary spasms in the muscles affecting the bowel area are probably the most common causes of such incontinence. Sensation may be reduced in the bowel area and you may not be aware that there has been a build-up of faecal material, until an involuntary movement of the anal sphincter occurs. Prior constipation might lead to this build-up and release of faecal material, as well as a lack of coordination in the muscles controlling bowel movements.

Although constipation and bowel incontinence may look like two separate problems, often they may be linked, so initially it is a good idea to try similar management. This involves establishing what is often known technically as a *bowel regimen*. In addition to checking your diet, as suggested in response to the question on constipation, making a regular time of day in which you try and have a bowel movement can be very helpful. This 'retraining' is not an easy task and may take some weeks or even months to achieve, but there is some evidence that it can reduce both constipation and bowel incontinence.

You can undergo some complex tests for difficult problems with bowel incontinence, but there are relatively few specialist centres to assess and help manage these problems. For most people with MS, a tried and tested combination of everyday techniques will probably be a good first step.

8
Pain and sensations

Changes in sensation

**I sometimes get pins and needles and occasionally a
burning sensation in my legs. What is happening?**

These symptoms are very likely due to MS. You may get them in
other parts of your body as well. After exercise, or at night, this
pain may get worse. The sensation of **pins and needles** commonly occurs with the interruption and resumption of nerve signals to particular areas of your body. Closely related sensations,
such as **tingling**, may also appear occasionally, as signals to and
from the affected area vary. Some people take tricyclic antidepressants if the sensations are associated with pain; burning
sensations have been treated with TENS (transcutaneous electrical nerve stimulation), a technique where a small portable
machine applies a tiny electric current to the area concerned.

**My hand has started to tremble when I go to pick
something up. How can I control this problem?**

Most people have some kind of *tremor* although it is usually so
slight that it is not seriously troubling. The most common type
experienced in MS is what is known as *action tremor*. The effect
of this kind of tremor is that the nearer your hand approaches
an object when reaching for it, the more your hand trembles, so
that it becomes difficult either to pick up or control an object –
such as a cup. Other kinds of tremor are much rarer. There are
really no drugs currently available that have been specifically

developed to assist tremor; drugs that have been tried often produce other unwanted effects. Drugs which are known as *beta-blockers*, such as propranolol, may have the most effect but, even so, they were originally developed for other purposes.

People tend to develop their own methods of coping with tremor. These include such things as:

- bracing an arm against a piece of furniture;

- making the arm immobile for a specific task;

- working out movements with a physiotherapist which are as smooth as possible;

- adding weights to an arm.

I have had a feeling of numbness quite frequently in my left arm, and then the other day on the right side of my face. Can I do anything about this?

Numbness is quite a common sensory symptom in MS and is due to inflammation or damage to your nerves. Your feet or hands, and also your legs and arms, the lower body itself and parts of the face can also sometimes be affected. Numbness in the hands makes it difficult to hold or pick things up, and can be worrying when things which are hot or sharp. You will have to use your sight more to recognize things: if the numbness is affecting your legs, you will need to check not only where, but how, you are walking.

Balance

I sometimes feel dizzy and have, on occasions, lost my balance. I don't want people to think I am drunk. Can I do anything about it?

From a social point of view this is one of the most difficult issues to manage. Loss of balance is basically a problem caused by damage to part of the brain, and dizziness tends to be caused by damage to the middle ear (*vestibular system*). The problem can be worse if you have spasticity or weakness in your legs. Walking aids (perhaps a stick or crutches) will help you avoid some painful falls that might occur. Using such aids will bring social benefits at least, signalling to others that you are not drunk, but that you have some physical problems with movement.

Dizziness (*vertigo*) often disappears of its own accord. Steroids can help, if the dizziness is both acute and persistent, or sometimes diazepam (Valium). There is one other apparently strange method which may help: when the vertigo feels worse on moving, it can often be helped by exaggerating those movements. Deliberately falling on to a bed (or other very soft surface) on your left and right side, and backwards, three times each way, may 'rebalance' the vestibular system, at least temporarily. You may also find that there is a particular position that lessens the vertigo, say being on one side rather than the other.

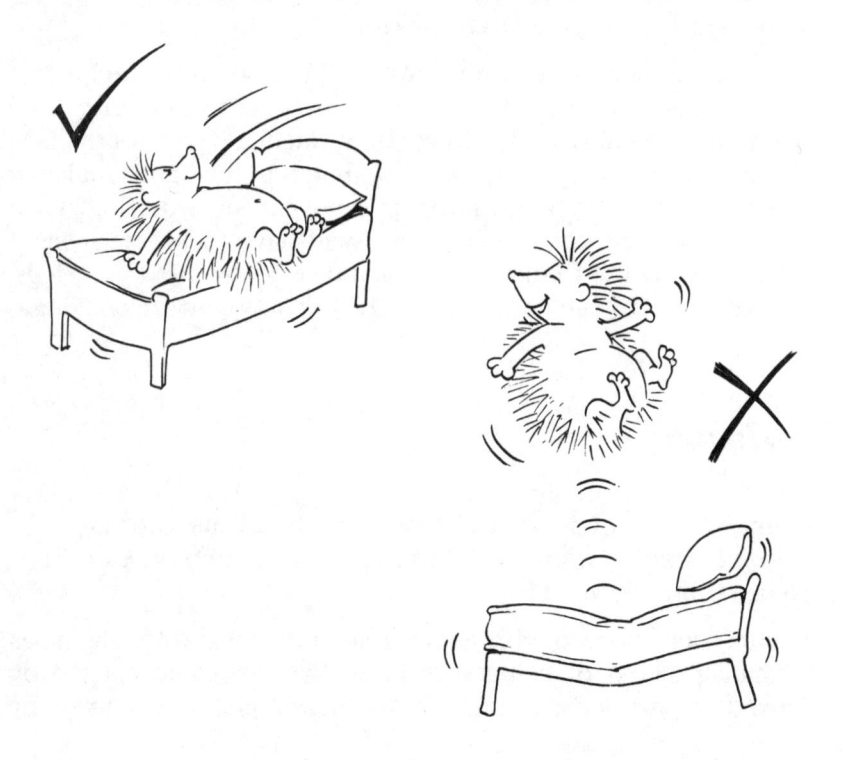

Pain and spasticity

Following my diagnosis with MS, I have started experiencing some pain and tightness in my chest. Climbing stairs can really wind me. Should I bother my doctor, and what can be done about it?

It is very important to understand that you, just like anyone else, can become ill from conditions other than MS itself; not every twinge, pain or symptom results from the MS. What you describe may, of course, be nothing serious, but the symptoms could indicate hypertension (raised blood pressure) or be signs of heart disease. Current research and clinical knowledge indicate that the symptoms you describe are not those of MS – if they persist then you must consult your GP. The same advice applies to other signs and symptoms that might indicate the presence of conditions unrelated to MS.

I often get what seem to be cramps or spasms in my legs. My legs quite often go rigid, and the cramps are very painful, making my life really difficult. What can I do?

What you are describing is known medically as spasticity, in which control of your muscles is affected in a particular way following damage by MS to the CNS. In effect, several muscles are contracting simultaneously, both those which assist a particular movement and those which would normally counter it. This is quite a common symptom in MS: it can occur in the calf, thigh or buttock area, as well as the arms and, occasionally, the lower back. Make sure you see your doctor, because spasticity can lead to *contractures*, where the muscle shortens, making the symptom worse.

Exercise, such as swimming, is one of the best ways of managing this spasticity. There are drugs to help as well. One of the most common and widely used is baclofen (Lioresal), which is often very effective but can have side effects; some people find it hard to tolerate high doses. Other muscle relaxants, such as the widely used diazepam (Valium), can also be used, but may have general sedative effects, causing drowsiness. Some newer drugs include dantrolene (Dantrium) and tizanidine (Zanaflex).

I seem to be getting several aches and pains in various parts of my body. Are these linked to my MS?

People with MS have known for many years that specific symptoms can cause considerable pain, and this is now being recognized. Chronic pain is experienced by about 50% of people with MS and almost everyone will experience some kind of pain at some point. The pain that you are talking about is almost certainly caused by cramps in your muscles. It can usually be controlled through muscle-relaxing drugs, such as baclofen (Lioresal) (see the question above).

Some people experience what is known as *trigeminal neuralgia*, in the form of facial pain. Drug treatment for this includes carbamazepine (Tegretol), and steroid therapy for the inflammation. Temporomandibular joint (TMJ) pain affects the jaw area, and you may get more general migraine or tension headaches. Drug therapy can help, but the cause of the pain should be investigated first, and particularly the extent to which it is linked to MS, or to some other cause. Don't forget that not all pains are caused by the disease!

I find the heat a big problem; not only does my MS get worse, but I also get a lot of pain. Why is this?

MS sufferers do find heat a problem. Heat, particularly enhanced body heat, changes the process of nerve conduction, and may result in the sensation of weak muscles and limbs. Heat can also exacerbate other symptoms, such as pain associated with inefficient nerve transmission. Conversely, when the core body temperature is cooler, nerve conduction and muscle function appear to be better, particularly in MS. So try and avoid situations, including vigorous exercise, where your core body temperature is raised.

9
Fatigue, cognitive and mental problems, and depression

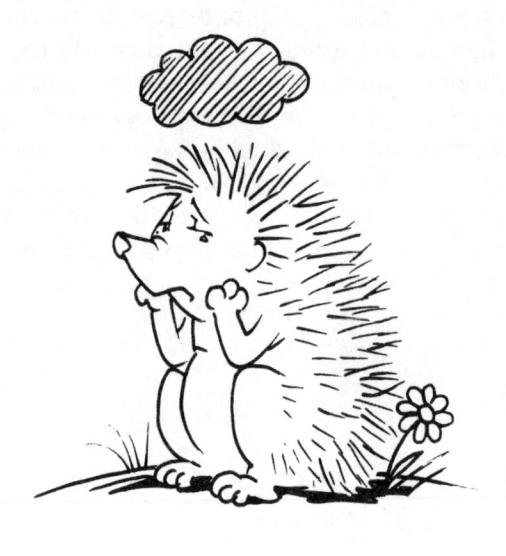

Fatigue or tiredness is one of the most debilitating symptom of MS and one that worries many people. Some ideas for management of fatigue are given here.

Research has identified two broad areas where MS seems to be involved or has effects that are not so much to do with the mind in general, but with what are more neatly and technically considered as cognitive issues on the one hand, and attitudinal and emotional issues on the other.

Cognitive issues are those which concern our thinking, memory and other skills that we use to form and understand language; how we learn and remember things; how we process information; how we plan and carry out tasks; how we recognize objects, and how we calculate. It was thought until recently that memory loss and some other cognitive problems were a rare occurrence. However, more recent research has suggested that a range of cognitive problems varying widely in type and severity may be present in many people with MS.

As far as emotional and attitudinal issues in MS are concerned, early research suggested that some people were emotionally *labile* (meaning their emotions fluctuated rapidly), and that other variable emotional symptoms or states arose which appeared to be specific to people with the disease. However, it proved difficult to tell whether the problems were a personal – indeed an emotional – reaction to the onset of MS, or were caused by the MS itself. Current research is indicating that there are problems of an emotional kind that might be linked to the disease itself, as well as personal reactions to it.

Fatigue

**The worst symptom of my MS seems to be this fatigue.
I feel I can hardly do anything. Not only that, it seems to
come when I least expect it. What is it?**

Up to 90% of people with MS experience major tiredness or what they often feel is a much more overwhelming feeling, which they call **fatigue**, often on a daily basis. Some types of fatigue may be explicable, even if it is overwhelming, in that it occurs during or after even modest exercise, or activity of some kind, when frequent breaks to recover and continue are needed. However, there is another kind of fatigue which many people experience and that is almost absolute exhaustion, where they can do nothing, other than rest immediately. On many occasions this fatigue seems to come out of nowhere just as you describe.

Fatigue in MS is often uniquely associated with heat (or being hot) (see Chapter 8). It is not linked closely with age, or degree of disability or, indeed, any particular type of MS. Many everyday activities may bring on, or be associated with, fatigue, but it does appear to be linked to a greater or lesser degree with:

- doing things – using motor skills, or being mobile;

- sleep disturbances;

- particular mood states (such as depression – see later section);

- some cognitive problems that may occur in MS (see Chapter 9).

At present there is no one known cause of fatigue in MS. Possible explanations have ranged from links with:

- immune dysfunction;

- problems associated with muscular control and movement (resulting in badly conditioned muscles and muscle activity);

- pre-existing or subsequently acquired psychological states, making the fatigue worse.

Is there anything I can do to help it?

Understandably, as the specific cause of MS fatigue is not known, the means of managing it tend to be related to the circumstances in which it occurs, and to control it we use what appears to work. Initially, it is important that your symptom is recognized as genuine by medical and other health care staff; this has not always happened. However, you will probably have to manage much of the day-to-day aspects of fatigue yourself, for drug therapies (see below) are often only partially successful.

You will, of necessity, have worked out some ways of managing your fatigue, such as identifying activities that appear to precede the fatigue and avoiding them whenever possible. You might not be able to do this every time, and many people develop 'pacing' strategies, trying to work intermittently with rest periods, or use some other ways of relaxing during the day. Often the fatigue seems to be related to particular times of the day, and you could focus your activities earlier or later than this period. You could try longer term 'pacing' too, trying to balance activities over periods of days or weeks. People with MS may do something that they enjoy or indeed have to do, knowing that they will have a couple of 'bad fatigue days' following this activity. However, 'fatigue management strategy' tends to be a complicated business, taking a lot of energy in itself to think through all the permutations that might occur.

On another front, there is currently considerable interest in various non-drug-based approaches to MS fatigue. General professional support is important, and a range of strategies may be offered. Specific and carefully planned exercise programmes have been found to reduce feelings of fatigue, but only temporarily (see next section). Behavioural therapy can help to alleviate other psychological symptoms that might exacerbate the fatigue, but these non-drug professional approaches have not been successful so far for most people with MS over the medium and longer term.

Some drugs have helped, the two most well known being magnesium pemoline (Cylert), which stimulates the central nervous system (CNS), and amantadine hydrochloride (amantadine; Symmetrel), an antiviral agent. Another line of attack is to try some antidepressants, particularly those which have a low sedative effect, for they may help the tiredness even if you are not clinically depressed. Beta-interferon drugs may have some effect on fatigue if, indeed, they help the immune system.

So for now, you will probably best manage your fatigue through your own lifestyle adjustments, with occasional help from drugs such as amantadine. Much more research is needed on this issue, especially as it worries so many people with MS.

Cognitive and mental problems

I have always thought that MS was a disease that affected various parts of your body, but where your mind wasn't affected at all. Am I wrong? Do people with MS also suffer from mental illness and premature dementia?

First of all we just need to clarify what you mean by 'mind'. People mean all sorts of things by 'mind': it can cover their thoughts, feelings and emotions, and often their spiritual life – in the sense of the 'meaning' that they make of their own lives, and indeed of all life. Thus there is a pretty broad set of issues raised here. Another issue raised in your question is whether the MS itself causes problems in the mind through its physical onset or progression, or whether the reactions of people with MS, emotional or otherwise, to the disease lead to any such problems.

Whilst we are not trying to be evasive, this question does need a slightly complicated answer. MS does not itself cause 'dementia' or, in the broadest sense, mental illness. Of course people with MS, just like anyone else of a similar age and sex, can suffer mental illness or dementia, but they do not appear to suffer these more frequently than anyone else.

However, clinically, people with MS do appear to have more **depression** (see next section) compared to other people, and perhaps have what might be called **mood swings** rather more often. More recently, studies have shown that many people with MS have some problems with memory and with what are called their *cognitive abilities*, and these seem to be associated with the effects of the disease. Nevertheless, many people do not think of depression, or for that matter mood swings, as mental illnesses; the cognitive difficulties that many people with MS may have are different from, and have a completely different cause and course to, those for dementia. We discuss depression and mood swings later in this chapter.

Why is memory and thinking affected in MS?

This issue is now being explored in great detail, but there are still many puzzles remaining. Whether you will develop cognitive problems cannot be predicted in any precise way. Little relationship has been found between physical disability and cognitive problems, or between the latter and disease duration, even when there are few sensory or mobility problems. However, there does seem to be a relationship between the number of lesions or plaques caused by MS in the relevant areas of the brain and the extent of cognitive performance, but at present it is difficult to pin the relationship down precisely enough, so that any cognitive difficulties can be predicted. However, there is substantial research under way at present using the latest imaging technologies –magnetic resonance imaging (MRI), for example – to locate and picture the areas of the brain affected by MS, and to link this data to more sophisticated neuropsychological tests for cognitive difficulties.

How will I know whether I have some cognitive problems?

This is not as simple a question as it sounds. It may be quite difficult for you to judge yourself whether you have problems with your memory or thinking. A number of studies have shown that other people (particularly family or household members) may be able to make a better judgement about these issues than you. This is not surprising for, in many aspects of our daily life, we can all change without necessarily realizing the nature or extent of that change – until someone tells us.

Nevertheless, there are different issues involved here in acknowledging, understanding and managing these kinds of problems. Sometimes people with MS may be so depressed or anxious that they think their cognitive problems are worse than in fact they are; on the other hand, they may not want to acknowledge them at all, for they do not want to think that MS may affect their cognitive as well as their physical functions. Although we have mentioned that family perceptions may be more accurate on occasions, they may be interpreted in other ways. They may not be seen as effects of the MS, but as indications that you are trying to get out of your fair share of work or responsibility. Although we all suffer from memory lapses from time to time, it may be tempting for you or some family members to put down every piece of forgetfulness to the MS. To avoid possible uncertainties, concerns or perhaps even recriminations, you should seek an objective assessment of any cognitive problems, if possible with a referral usually from your neurologist.

Will my cognitive problems get worse?

It is difficult to tell. We have noted how hard it is to predict these problems already. For most people, as far as we can judge, cognitive performance is likely to be reasonably stable for long periods of time, although for a few people it may worsen more rapidly; however, even if one of the functions gets worse, others may stay the same. Since we believe that cognitive functions may remain more stable than some other symptoms of MS, then it is possibly even more worthwhile to investigate ways of dealing with them, for any strategies you employ may continue to be used over a long period of time.

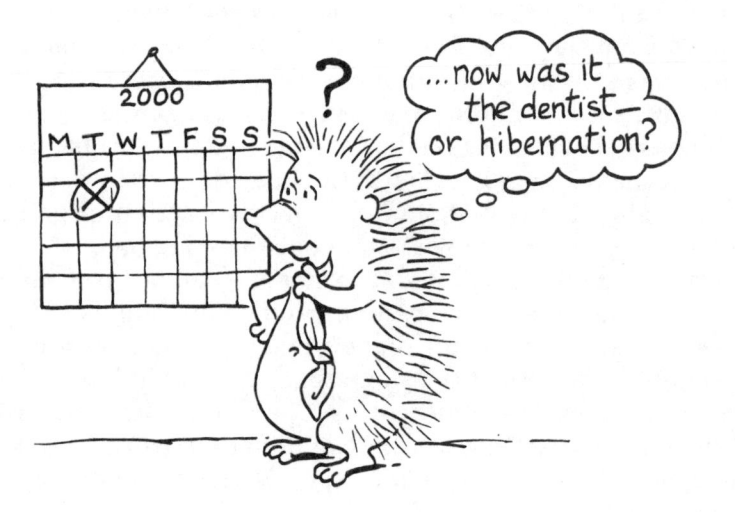

Are there any drugs I can take to help my memory or concentration?

At present there are no drugs approved and accepted for the management of such problems as memory or concentration in MS. Memory problems are, of course, not limited to people with MS, and there is considerable research in this area. However, the cause of memory problems varies between different conditions, so drugs that might be helpful for people with Alzheimer's disease, who have very severe memory problems, would not necessarily be useful for people with MS. Nevertheless, there is increasing research to see whether a number of drugs, often originally developed for other purposes, might help people with MS, but it may be some time before they are proved to be of value and become widely available.

You have said that people with MS may have cognitive problems. I think my memory is going and I have problems concentrating. If there are no drugs to help, what can I do to help myself?

People with MS can be affected by a range of cognitive prob-lems, and it is difficult to advise you precisely without knowing exactly what they are. The difficulties that you mention specifi-cally – memory and concentration – are quite common.

As far as the **concentration** goes, everyone has occasional problems concentrating on things. Sometimes the problem is that we have many things going on at the same time – television, other people talking and a whole range of other activities going on. However, for someone with MS, concentrating on one of these activities – a conversation, for example – can be quite difficult, when so much else is happening. So the key thing is to try and have only one thing going on at a time – a conversation or the television, not both at the same time. You might have to move between rooms to achieve this. Find out when and where problems for you are most difficult, and then work on reducing the distractions to the minimum. Obviously changing your pattern of normal activities to help you concentrate may not be easy, but may be preferable to having continuing communication problems.

As far as **memory** is concerned, there are many ways in which you can jog your memory. Some of these are routine, and may appear overpedantic or fussy for someone who has only minor memory difficulties, but all help to deal with short-term memory problems. For example, just making sure that clocks and watches show the right time; ensuring that today's date is prominently displayed somewhere; having a message board to note activities for today and tomorrow; having a list of activities that you are intending to do, with times and dates, perhaps in the form of a diary or similar record. Although this might seem almost too formal, note things down that you have agreed to do, or that you and others think important, so that it doesn't appear that you have forgotten it.

My husband sometimes 'loses the plot' when he is speaking to me. We both find it difficult to deal with. Is there anything I can do?

One of the first things is to ensure that there are as few distractions as possible. For example, make sure that children aren't demanding attention, or that a television is off, because such distractions can cause the loss of a train of thought. It is also possible that his train of thought is fine, but he finds it difficult to form the words because of problems in the muscular control of his speech. In this case, it is a question of both of you being patient.

You could remind him where he has got to in the conversation, so that it gives both a cue to him, and time for the words to come. However, it may be rather very frustrating for him if you 'put words into his mouth'; this can easily happen if you are busy, so try and arrange in advance times when you can have a quiet and reasonably distraction-free conversation.

Depression

I am worried about depression and MS. I have recently been diagnosed, and have heard that depression is very common in MS. Is this the case?

The incidence of depression amongst people with MS has been a matter of controversy for many years. In the early years of research it was thought that relatively few people with the condition had 'clinical' depression, but more recent research indicates that the level of depression is far higher than was previously thought.

Of course one of the problems is what you mean by the term 'depression'. It is a word used often in everyday conversation, as things don't go as we would like them to. If these sorts of feelings are relatively transient, and go away without any major consequences for how we live our lives, then we probably do not need any professional help.

However, more serious depression, i.e. what we might technically call a *major depressive episode*, is likely to be associated with a whole series of changes to everyday life. For example, we may:

- lose our appetite;

- have serious sleep problems;

- feel that life is hopeless;

- generally think that we are worthless; and even

- entertain suicidal thoughts occasionally.

Recent research suggests that up to 50% of people with MS (compared to only 5–15% of people without) will experience one or more of these episodes at some point in their lives, and at any one time perhaps one in seven may be experiencing this kind of depression.

Although it may not be easy for either you or your doctor to distinguish depression in this more serious form from some of the other symptoms and problems of MS (since sleep disturbance, fatigue and difficulty in concentrating may be associated with other consequences of the condition), it is best to aware of it.

Why do people with MS have such a high rate of depression?

At present it is difficult to give an answer to this question. A very well designed study investigating the life-time risk of major depression in MS found no genetic basis for this high level – near relatives of people with MS actually had a lower risk of developing depression than other people. No link was found with damage to specific parts of the brain or central nervous system, or with the severity of damage, although it is still possible that certain kinds of nervous system damage in MS may produce an increased risk of depression.

Overall, at present it seems likely that the other factors influencing the development of depression are to do with people themselves: their situation, sometimes called their 'coping style' in dealing with the MS, and the kind of support that they have from relatives and friends. Of course, it would be expected that having a serious neurological condition, often relatively early in adulthood, would produce feelings of sadness, grief and major concern about the future. The question from a clinical – and indeed personal point of view – is when and on what basis these feelings and concerns turn into major depression. No one has an easy or simple answer to this at the moment.

I really can't think of the future at all with my MS. I just seem to be living for the present.

Something like MS is likely to cast a shadow over what the future might bring, particularly as MS affects young adults. Of course, most people will not achieve all the dreams they may have had, but they only realize this afterwards. With MS you have to be more realistic much earlier, and the possibilities seem more limited than those of others. The important thing is to be **realistic**, **not over-pessimistic** about the future. There could be many possibilities open to you, and indeed, as many people with

MS have shown, many personal dreams that can be fulfilled. It may help to talk some of these over with a good friend, or perhaps a counsellor.

Mood swings and euphoria

My wife says that I have dreadful mood swings. I know that this upsets her. Is it my MS that is causing this?

The cause of these is still very much under debate, but recognizing that mood swings exist is the first step in being able to manage them more effectively. If you have what can be referred to medically as a *bipolar disorder* with relatively rapid and severe swings between depression and elation, you should seek medical assistance.

Some people experience an 'elevation of mood'. This is now often described as *euphoria* and can be linked with mood swings. Less attention has been paid to the much more serious problem of depression. It is possible that, in some people with MS, a euphoric presentation has cloaked an underlying depression. Euphoria has been viewed as a widespread phenomenon partly because of the very positive reactions – the relief almost – that some people with MS feel once diagnosed. Because the process, and then the communication, of a diagnosis may take some time (see Chapter 4), some people feel that their symptoms may have been due to even more serious conditions – a brain tumour, for example, or that they were 'going mad'. Some doctors have treated the, often profound, relief of some of their patients on hearing that they 'only' have MS, as indicating a euphoric state caused by the MS, rather than an understandable relief that they have a condition far less threatening than others they had feared.

The particular phenomenon of 'euphoria' at the time of diagnosis seems to be overemphasized and, in terms of everyday symptom management, other emotional problems, particularly those centred around depression, are more harmful and significant. However, inappropriate laughter and other related signs of a kind of euphoria (which may occur as the MS progresses) may occasionally be embarrassing and should be considered seriously with assessment and support.

I am worried that I seem to break into tears very easily, or laugh almost uncontrollably at times. My husband is very concerned, as indeed I am. Is there anything I can do about this?

It is difficult to give you a precise reason why this problem occurs. Indeed there may be several causes.

In general, people with different social circumstances and backgrounds may have very different approaches to the expression of emotion. For example, some emotional behaviour, that you may personally feel inappropriate to you and to people whom you know, may be entirely acceptable to other people. Regarding your situation now, what is or was normal for you, your family and friends, has been changed by the different ways in which you are expressing yourself. Particularly in our relatively emotionally restrained British society, any outward expression of emotion might be considered abnormal, and this could make your situation and that of your husband more difficult.

However, there could be a number of other issues here. The emotion you feel and express may be entirely appropriate but – in social terms – exaggerated. Here your emotional response is just rather 'too strong' for the particular situation. You could try breathing deeply, pausing before the tears or laughter come, particularly in stressful situations. If you find yourself laughing or crying without any apparent cause – indeed your mood may be totally at variance with this expression of emotion – and it is difficult to stop, almost certainly this is a result of damage caused by MS itself, probably to areas of the brain controlling the release of emotional expression. This problem has to be managed socially, which is not an easy task, but you could be prescribed medications which have some dampening effect on the release of emotions. It would be best to consult your GP or neurologist about these matters.

10
Mobility

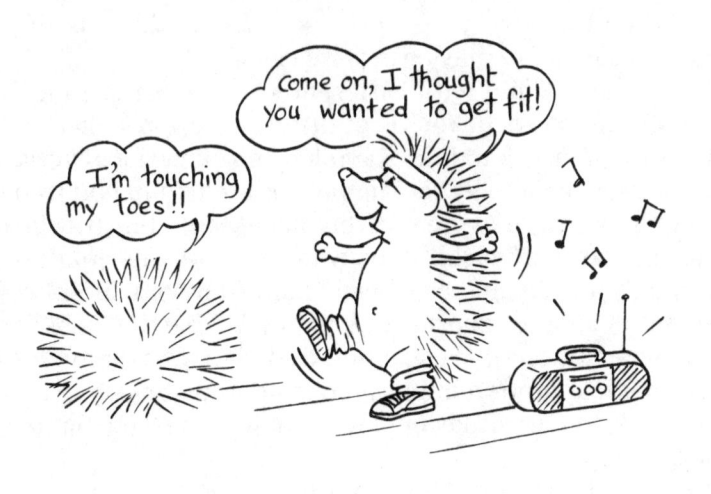

One of the first things that many people notice with MS is that they sometimes have problems of movement in their arms or legs, or in other parts of the body and often in due course, this happens more continuously. The reasons for this are clear. Damage to various sites in the central nervous system (CNS) from MS leads to a loss of control, or only partial control, of the relevant groups of muscles. However, mobility or movement problems can be very variable, both from person to person, and over time in one person, depending on the overall disease development, and on whether you are currently in the middle of an attack or in remission. The main concern in terms of management is to maintain as much mobility as possible, in particular to avoid what might be called 'secondary' damage in the form of wasting (atrophied) muscles, which occurs as a result of prolonged lack of use. Of course, it is important for both you, and for those involved in caring for or supporting you, to know why you have movement problems, and to tailor any exercise and management programmes to these problems.

Exercises

I have been told to do specific exercises for my MS. Why is this?

The body has many muscles in many unexpected places. Even people without MS, especially if they are not undergoing comprehensive physical training, find that unusual or different forms of exercise leave them with aching or stiff muscles because they are unused to exercise. In the case of people with MS, they have the additional problem that more of their muscles may become underused through specific damage to the nervous system. So the main aim of exercising is to:

- try and keep as many muscles as possible in good working order;
- strengthen those that have become weak;
- help keep joints mobile;
- help prevent them from getting stiff;
- help your coordination and balance;
- improve your circulation – and in doing so help other body functions;
- help reduce spasticity in more advanced MS;
- help prevent pressure sores (for sites of common pressure sores see Figure 10.1).

Overall, one could say that exercise will help you maintain your maximum independence. Some floor and chair exercises are shown in Figures 10.2 and 10.3.

What professional help is available?

Although there has been an explosion of health and fitness clubs, which might be thought to help people with mobility or other similar difficulties, very few of them have staff who will be aware of MS and its effects on movement. So it's a good idea to seek the help of members of the key profession dealing with mobility and movement problems, and that is **physiotherapy**. Normally you

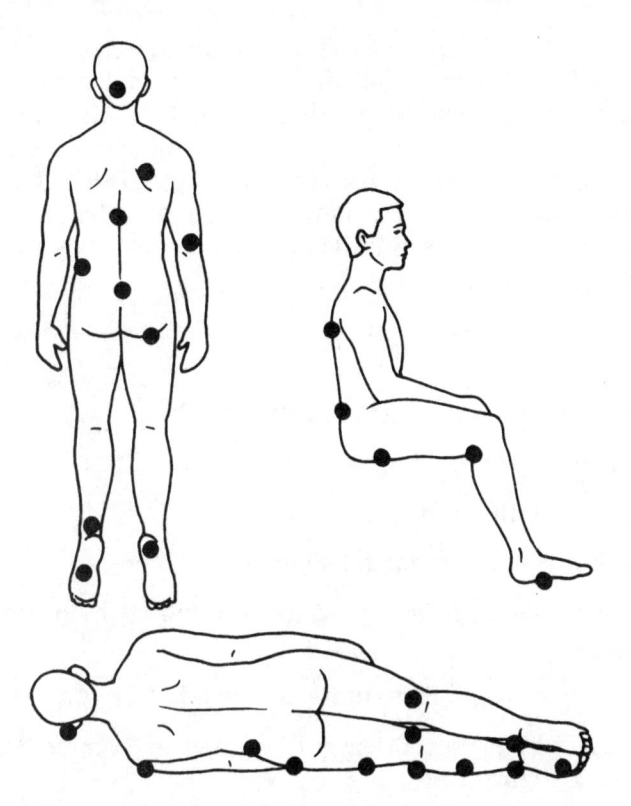

Figure 10.1 Areas where pressure sores can develop.

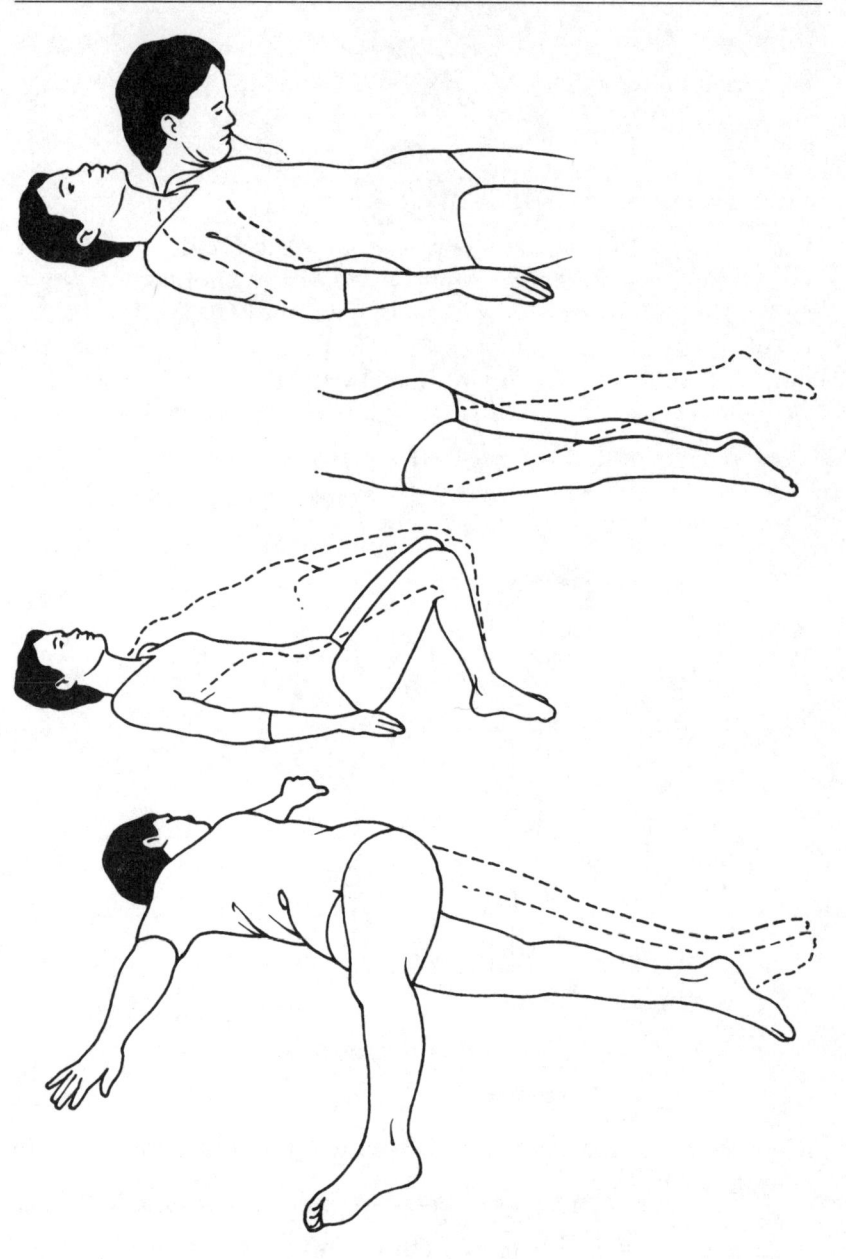

Figure 10.2 Floor exercises.

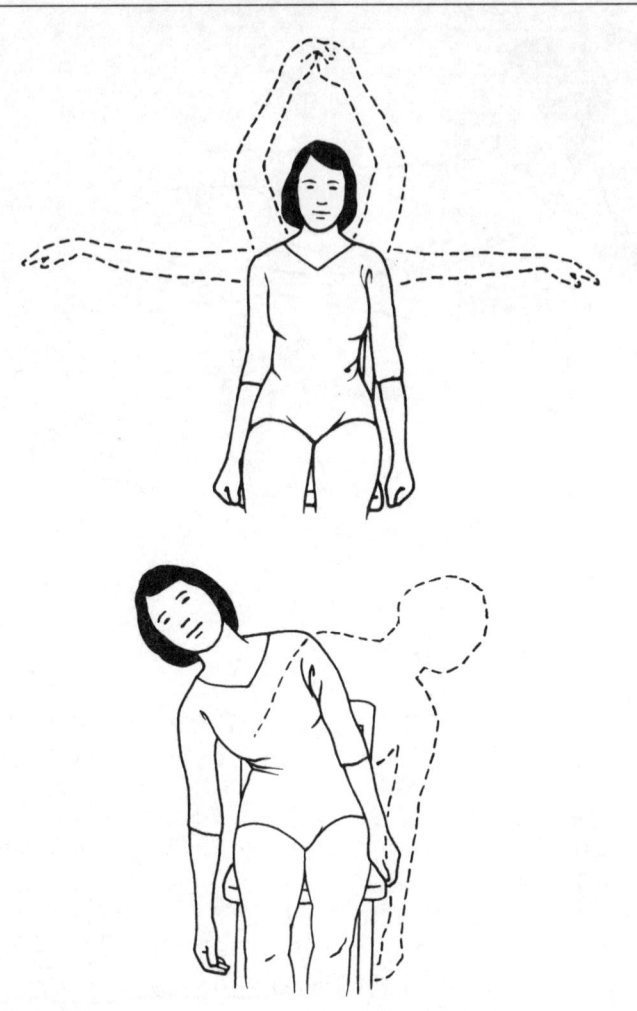

Figure 10.3 Chair exercises.

will be referred for a consultation with a physiotherapist by your neurologist or GP.

Most physiotherapists until relatively recently have been largely concerned with acute injuries, in which a return to full, or reasonably full, functioning can be anticipated. Relatively few

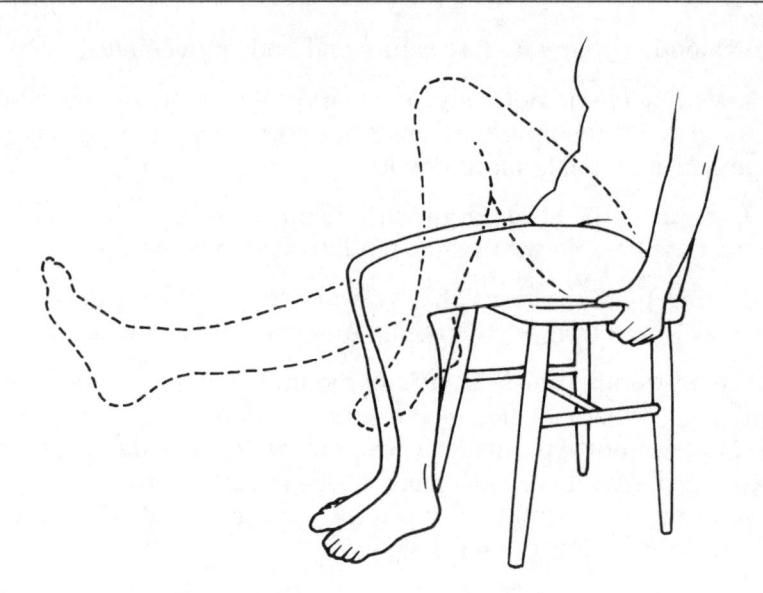

Figure 10.3 Chair exercises (continued).

were specialized in longer term chronic conditions like MS, in which the main aims are to slow down deterioration, or to try and maintain existing function. So, until recently, many physiotherapists have not fully understood MS or its problems, and how to manage it effectively – even if they were technically well trained in other respects. This situation is changing rapidly through the activities of the MS Society, the establishment of specialist training programmes and courses, and a general realization of the value of physiotherapy for people with MS. However, you should check, either with your referring doctor or with the physiotherapist, that they have had experience of managing people with MS.

How will a physiotherapist evaluate my movement problems? Will any exercises be recommended?

A physiotherapist will normally undertake a number of assessments of your movement ability. These would include generally:

- evaluating your general posture and body movements;

- taking account not only of what you can do in the clinic, surgery or hospital, but also what problems you may have in and around the home and work;

- measuring the strength of various muscles, as well as assessing how flexible your joints, tendons and muscles are;

- testing the sensations that you may have in or around your muscles, as well as your ability to sense cold and heat.

Some physiotherapists, particularly in leading hospitals, may undertake what is called *gait analysis*, i.e. a formal assessment of how you move, particularly how you walk, investigating things like speed, rhythm of movement, stride and step length.

A number of different types of exercise might be recommended depending on this diagnosis.

- For your overall fitness, **general exercises** may be recommended, not necessarily linked to any particular movement symptom of your MS.

- **Exercises to improve your *cardiovascular* fitness** will increase your heart rate, and are good for your circulation.

- **Stretching exercises** will decrease the risk of spasticity and contractures. These exercises work by stretching muscles and tendons to increase their flexibility and elasticity.

- **Resistance exercises**, with the use of weights or other devices, help increase the strength of muscles that have been weakened.

- **Range of motion exercises** focus on improving the degree of motion of joints in the body, and aim to overcome, as far as possible, difficulties caused by stiffness in joints or problems in tendons and ligaments.

Are there any exercises I should not do if I have MS?

There are no intrinsically harmful exercises for people with MS. It is a question about how and when you do exercises, rather than whether you ought to do them. For the most part, the main problems are related to getting overheated or exhausted, which we have noted elsewhere may on occasion lead to a temporary increase in some MS symptoms (see Chapter 8). Your own commonsense will normally tell you when you are exerting yourself too much. Generally, if you exercise carefully and regularly, with periodic breaks, you should find that you can get the most reward from the exercise.

My wife has MS. Are there any special things that I should do or avoid doing when I help her with the exercises recommended by the physiotherapist?

In general, the physiotherapist should have indicated how you can help your wife but, apart from following those instructions carefully, the following broad points may assist you.

- First encourage her to undertake as much movement as possible, but try to avoid impeding her movements.

- When you are grasping one of her limbs, use as even a pressure as possible with the whole of your hand, and perform your movements as smoothly as you can, helping her to perform a passive exercise (an exercise undertaken with/on a person by another person).

- Don't apply increased pressure at the most extreme points of the movement and, if a spasm occurs when you touch a limb, wait to see whether the spasm ceases and then, if it does, continue to assist as long as the movement is comfortable for her.

Thinking generally, what broad guidelines would you offer about exercise and movement for someone with MS?

Most of the guidelines are quite sensible if you think about them.

- Try and undertake those exercises that you have been recommended to do by a physiotherapist regularly, preferably every day – unless the physiotherapist indicates otherwise.

- Whether you have been given advice by a physiotherapist or not, it would be wise to try and move around as much as you can, and to sit and stand as erect as possible.

- Try to exercise within your own capacity, i.e. do not get over-tired, and try not to worry if you perform less well on a bad day. Everybody's performance varies from day to day.

- Also try and recognize when you need professional advice about problems that you are experiencing and that are not being helped by your current pattern of exercises.

Although I know that I must do exercises, my MS fatigue prevents me from doing them. What can I do?

This is a difficult problem for many people with MS, who may feel they are tired for much of the time. The key to solving this problem may be working out ways in which you can take advantage of the times when you feel less fatigued in order to do modest but well-targeted exercise. Look carefully at the day-to-day activities you undertake, to see whether they might be rearranged and result in less fatigue. Sometimes, introducing rest periods and using specific aids for certain activities will result in less fatigue, and the chance to undertake limited and helpful exercises. You may also need, perhaps in consultation with a physiotherapist, to review the exercises to make them less vigorous. After all, it is not only a question of getting your exercise regimen right, but of getting a good balance between exercise and relaxation as well.

I keep being told that posture is important. Why is this so?

Perhaps surprisingly, posture is one of the key things that affects how you feel, and in the slightly longer run affects various key pointers of your health. Many people, not just people with MS, have bad posture, in the sense that they do not stand or sit in ways that are good for their health; but for people with MS, especially where they are less active or, even worse, sitting for most of the day, the consequences of bad posture can be particularly worrying. Posture, which relates to many parts of your body, affects not only the way you look but, when it is bad, may produce muscle and joint strains, and secondary back problems. Furthermore, bad posture in a wheelchair or other chair may have more profound constrictive effects on your breathing and chest and other areas. This is why there is so much emphasis on standing or sitting in as upright a position as possible, and trying to ensure continuing flexibility in your joints and muscles to enable you to keep a good posture.

I have weakness in my legs and problems with my balance. Can exercise help in these areas?

Physiotherapy, or exercise in general, cannot remedy neurological problems, in the sense that exercise cannot 'mend' the damaged nerve fibres that lead to less effective control of muscles. Weakness in the legs, and problems of balance, may directly occur as a result of less effective nerve conduction, but there may be other (subsidiary) causes of both, that could be assisted by exercise. Try and find out, with advice from your neurologist or physiotherapist, the likely causes of these problems, and then with their help devise a programme of exercise therapy that takes account of the balance between neurological or other causes. You want to be certain that any special exercises that you do undertake, e.g. resistance exercises through using weights, are in fact likely to help you.

Problems with balance, particularly in MS, are very likely to be caused by damage to the relevant parts of your nervous system and are thus not remediable through exercise. However, additional problems can be caused by weakness or stiffness in the muscles and joints of the legs, and these may respond to a dedicated exercise programme.

Quite often my muscles in my leg contract and go rigid; I believe this is called 'spasticity'. I can't move and it's very painful. What can I do?

This is quite a common problem with MS, and can be awkward to deal with. Although the root cause lies in poor or inadequate signals via the spinal cord to muscles in the legs and elsewhere,

in general such problems are lessened if you have a regular programme of stretching and related exercises to help muscular
development, or at the very least to help prevent the muscles
wasting away. Ensure, as far as possible, that your joints, tendons and ligaments are as flexible as possible. You will also
know that there are certain positions in which spasticity is more
likely, and clearly these should be avoided. Try and keep your
head as central as possible when doing exercises and, if spasticity does occur, do a passive exercise as smoothly as possible to
relax your muscles. On occasion it has been found that towels
dipped in iced water and applied to the relevant area for a few
minutes at most may help the muscles to relax. Unfortunately, as
MS progresses, even with the most helpful exercise programme,
additional means – usually prescribed drugs – may be necessary
to assist the spasticity. You should consult your neurologist or
GP about the most relevant drugs.

**What about swimming as a way of getting some exercise,
even though I can't swim well and perhaps even less well
now that I have MS?**

Swimming is a good form of exercise for everyone, not just for
people with MS. However, it is especially helpful for you because
your bodyweight is supported by the water – the water will stabilize someone with balance problems. Weakened muscles can
operate in this environment and will strengthen from the resistance. In addition, as swimming involves many muscle systems
in your body, it can help to increase coordination.

   Your main practical problems may be issues such as where the
changing rooms are in relation to the pool, and obtaining
assistance to reach, and return from, the pool. You may also feel
self-conscious, as swimming involves people revealing more of
their bodies than in other activities – and you may be particularly
concerned about how you look or how you move amongst people
without MS. However, there are now more and more swimming
pools and leisure centres having special sessions for people with
disabilities, or those who need special help, and it might be worth
trying one of these sessions at first. If such sessions are not

available, try lobbying your local leisure centre/swimming pool for one. If neither of these options proves possible, it may still be worth asking whether there are quiet times of the day when the pool will be freer, and assistance is more likely to be available.

One point may prove to be important and that is the temperature of the water. The temperature that many people with MS find comfortable is about 30°C (86°F). Much lower temperatures appear to be too cold, although still tolerable, whereas much higher temperatures, often found in jacuzzis or spa baths, are sometimes associated with the onset of (temporary) MS symptoms. Also, in relation to your swimming activities, if you have troublesome bladder control, it may be worth discussing this with your neurologist or GP beforehand to try and ease your concerns.

I think something is happening to my left foot – it's no longer as straight as it was and it seems to have 'turned in'. What can I do?

There are several changes that may occur as a result of less effective nervous system control of your leg or ankle muscles. One of these problems is when your foot 'turns in' (*foot drop*) as a result of both the muscles and tendons on the inside of your foot becoming shorter, through underuse, than those on the outside of your foot. There are several ways of trying to remedy this – special braces and exercises, for example. Relevant exercises are crucial, undertaken both actively and passively. Indeed, the problem shows how important it is to undertake a preventative exercise programme at a very early stage, as it is for other potential mobility problems caused by MS.

Aids and equipment to assist with mobility and movement problems

Different tasks that most people deal with at home or when they are out include taking care of yourself, jobs in and around the house, and outside the house such as shopping – all these together are often called professionally *activities of daily living*. Although it is likely that you and members of your household will work out solutions to many of these tasks, occupational therapy is the profession which is mainly concerned with helping people to manage any difficulties they may have in daily living. You will almost certainly be offered a consultation with an occupational therapist (OT) at some point but, if you are not and want such professional advice, your GP or neurologist should be able to refer you to an OT to assist you. You also may need to use an occupational therapist if you wish to obtain aids and equipment through your local NHS Trust or Department of Social Services.

I am very unsteady on my legs, and I'm now afraid of falling in my house. What can I do?

Although you may be reaching the point where you need some sort of walking aid, there is quite a lot you can do to help yourself. First you should try and reduce the number of hazards in your home that might cause you to fall. For example, try and reduce or eliminate shiny, polished floors, loose rugs and mats, trailing electric cables, and other things left on the floor that you might trip over. Be careful of lively cats and dogs when you are moving around. Think carefully about how you arrange your furniture, so that you have a clear path where you usually walk and, for example, are not always confronted by a low coffee table when you move to the kitchen.

Falls often occur when you are getting in and out of chairs, so be careful and move as deliberately as you can (see Chapter 8). If you tend to use furniture for support when you move around the house, be very careful that you do not misjudge the distance to it, that it is stable enough to support you, and that it hasn't been moved since you last used it! Falls can easily result from problems like this. The trouble is that, after a while, you may get so used to using your furniture that, if you do take a slightly different route, you could be in difficulty!

In general, the key thing about moving around is to move slowly and deliberately, despite the urgent ringing telephone and the doorbell. For telephones, you really need an extension close to where you normally sit, and one or more where you can reach them relatively easily. For people who you know are coming to your door, or others who come regularly and who might need to contact you (such as the postman), you can let them know that it may take you a little time to get to the door. Other people will just have to wait!

It might be worth considering a personal alarm for use in emergencies – it will give you more reassurance. Of particular value are those systems which, at the press of button, will dial up a family member or someone else who could help you.

Housework is becoming a big problem not just because I have had to change so much to 'make it safe' for me, but partly because I can't actually do it all. What should I do?

Retaining even a very modest range of household activities is important, to feel that you are contributing to the household overall.

Rearrange the furniture and other things in the house as comfortably and safely as possible for yourself and others in your household. Other people in your household may want things in particular rooms, compared to where you feel you need them arranged for your safety, but you can probably come to a compromise over who arranges what room, as long as you have the minimum you need to be able to move around.

As far as tidying and cleaning goes, you are probably more conscious than others of this issue. Most of us are always about to clean or tidy something, and then leave it to the next day! There is a range of equipment that you can use from a standing position, or even at a distance from a sitting position, and these may allow you to do a little at a time, although the heavier jobs, and particularly those which involve moving around equipment – like vacuum cleaners – may need to be undertaken by others, unless you are very careful. You should be able to get further advice from your occupational therapist about available equipment and finding ways of managing to do at least some of the housework yourself.

I'm having increasing problems with getting in and out of my bath and also sitting down and getting up from the toilet. I find asking my husband to help me all the time rather undignified. What can I do?

Negotiating a bath requires both balance and strength, qualities that for some people with MS may be in short supply. There are several things that can be done in stages:

- Ensure that non-slip mats are both in the bath and on the floor and install grab bars at crucial points.

- It is good to have someone you can call if you do get into difficulty.

- Other options include bath seats and bath hoists.

- The larger types of shower will have sufficient space for a shower chair or bench to sit on and will be easier to access than a bath.

Although going to the toilet can be a problem for both sexes, many men in particular are not so used to helping others with such issues on an everyday basis.

A number of procedures can help. Velcro is useful as a fastener for trousers. If you have got limited or unsteady movement, you need to be very careful in lowering yourself on to the toilet. Stand directly in front of the seat, bend your knees until you can touch the sides of the seat with your hands, and then lower yourself down slowly. When raising yourself use the toilet seat to push yourself off. Check that the toilet seat is secure before you use it!

Adaptations to the toilet itself may be of help:

- Grab bars can be placed on adjacent walls if they are near enough.

- Where a toilet is standing away from a wall, you could consider an over-the-toilet adjustable frame which has arm-rests to help you raise and lower yourself.

- There is an increasingly wide range of commodes.

- You can install a slightly elevated toilet seat.

The number of different adaptations in this area is increasing rapidly, so consult your occupational therapist, or other sources of information about such products. See Figure 10.4 for ideas.

One of the most trying problems for people with MS is using toilet paper, for the manoeuvre involves considerable movement and dexterity. You might find a wet cloth more useful than toilet paper, or you might consider using a squeezy bottle full of

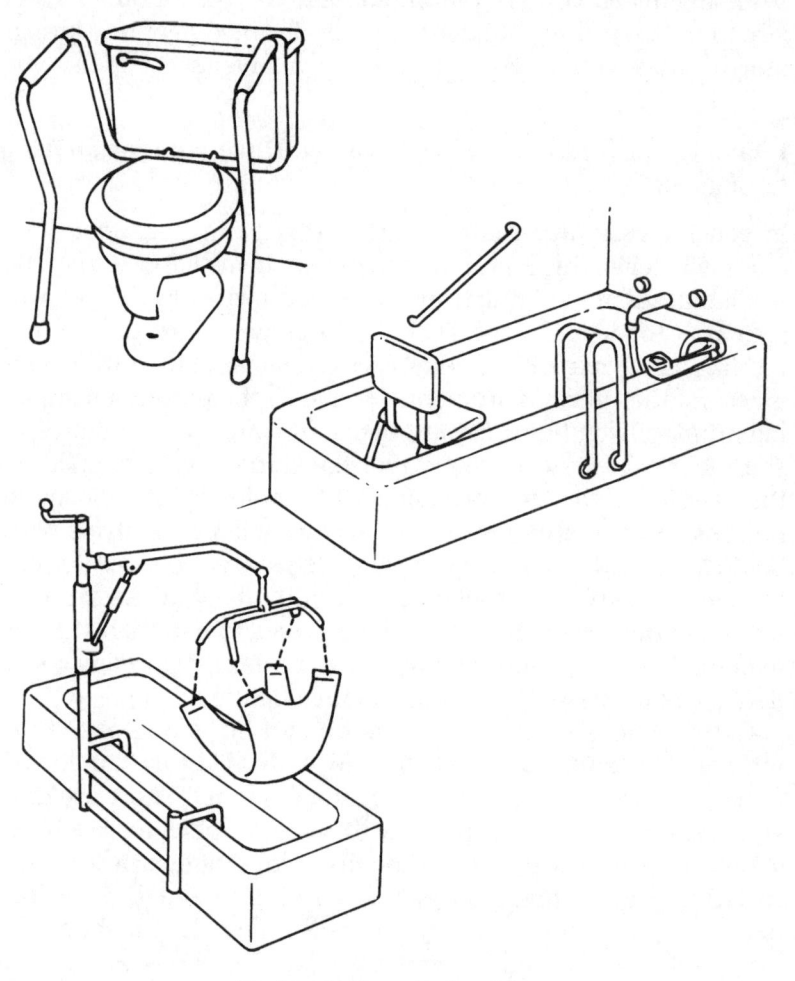

Fig 10.4 Bath and toilet aids.

(warm!) water. There is also special equipment, such as a toilet-paper holder, which could help. A bidet might be easier, although this may well not fit into your toilet area, can be rather expensive to install, and would need fitting to your water supply. Recently a portable toilet/bidet has been launched which might help people who are worried about travelling and having to deal with conventional, and therefore problematic, toilets elsewhere.

Finally, when you are out and about, you can obtain a special key from RADAR for public toilets for disabled people. More and more of these toilets are being made available (see Appendix 1).

I have general trouble with dressing. Have you got anything to suggest?

In general, tight-fitting clothes are harder to manage than looser ones, whatever the kinds of fixings on them. Large rather than small buttons are helpful; trousers or skirts with elasticated waists are easier to pull on or off. There is also now a wide range of dressing aids on the market including dressing sticks and button hooks.

One of the trickiest problems for men is the putting on and taking off of collars, ties and buttoned shirts. Most of the buttons on shirts can be left done up, so that the shirts can be slipped over the head or, if this is a problem, buttonholes can be closed, the buttons sewn on the outside of the shirt and Velcro strips placed behind them, so that when all the strips are closed it looks as though the shirt is buttoned in the traditional way. As far as ties are concerned, clip-on ones may be easier to use than the usual hand-tied ones or, alternatively, ties can be left already loosely tied and slipped over the head, and then tightened in place.

Getting shoes, socks and tights on and off is one of the most difficult problems for some people with MS, for it involves a range of movement, together with fine dexterity. There are different ways of coping with shoes. If you are able to reach your shoes, then there are Velcro shoe fastenings, and various devices to tighten laces, and you can learn single-handed tying techniques. If you cannot reach your shoes, then slip-on shoes are a better idea; you could convert your lace-up shoes into slip-ons with elastic laces, if the shoe tongue can be stitched into place.

Long-handled shoe horns will help you put on slip-on shoes and there are other aids available to help pull on (and take off) socks and tights – these usually work by gripping the socks or tights with the end of a hand-operated long-handled tool.

Working in the kitchen is now proving difficult. We are seriously wondering about whether we will have to redesign it, or whether a less drastic solution would help me manage food preparation and all the other things that I like to do in the kitchen.

If you are starting from scratch, or have decided on a major change in your kitchen area, then the main considerations are likely to be: accessibility, safety, ease of use, and whether other users of the area will be affected. Obviously the height of worktops and the sink area, especially if you are in a wheelchair, are important considerations. Think about access to and arrangements of cupboards, storage areas and cooking facilities, especially if you are likely to be carrying things from one place to another. Even if you are still relatively mobile, and not yet using a wheelchair, it would be sensible to think of future problems when you are making major changes – consider overhanging worktops, for example, so that they can be used from a seated position. Some kitchen systems allow for adjustment with changing circumstances: seek advice from your occupational therapist or specialist kitchen manufacturer about what is available for someone with your particular needs – now and for the future.

As regards food preparation, use foods which are pre-prepared in various forms, thus minimizing the amount of food preparation that you have to undertake. There has been a revolution in this area over the last few years, mainly owing to changing lifestyles, and the vastly increased number of women who work, both inside and outside the home. Many fresh foods that are harder for people with mobility problems to prepare – potatoes, salads, and vegetables, for example – can now all be purchased in pre-prepared form. Although there is an additional price to pay for these foods, and maybe a minor loss in nutrition, this is more than compensated for by the saving in time and energy that is

spent preparing everything yourself – just like most people without MS! The results – and indeed the process of cooking – of pre-
prepared foods can be just as enjoyable and challenging as
before. By using a combination of pre-prepared foods and some
that you have prepared yourself, you can put together innovative
meals. Try and phase what you do, so that you do not feel
exhausted from working overlong on single tasks without a
break. Look for special recipe books that not only suggest nutri-
tious foods, but also show short cuts in food preparation. If you
are worried about any nutritional issues, you should consult your
doctor, or ask for a referral to a dietitian or nutritionist.

Additional aids and equipment range from things like non-slip
mats to secure mixing bowls, high stools to work on, special trol-
leys, to padded handles to ensure a better grip. Everyday
kitchenware, such as knives, forks, spoons, ladles, and so on, are
now available in a form that will help you have a better grip, for
extra safety. You will quickly find those aids that help you most.
On the subject of safety, try and holds things with two hands, and
if you are carrying hot liquids, use containers with fitted lids.
Wearing rubber gloves can help.

Using a microwave oven, especially the modern combination
types, can be easier than a conventional one for some, and
although it can be seen as just another short cut, cooking interesting food in such an oven can be quite a challenge. One of the
additional benefits of a microwave oven is that it generates less
external heat than a conventional oven and, as many people with
MS find some of their symptoms get worse in heat, this is an
important advantage.

**I find I really can't use an ordinary pen or pencil any
more. Is there anything else that would help me?**

Fatter pens or pencils are becoming fashionable now because
they are ergonomically better for everyone's fingers. If your writing is a problem because of tremor, weight your wrist or use
weighted pens, etc., which may dampen down the tremor. There
are also various devices, writing guides for example, which help
you to form letters and words, lessening the effect of the tremor.

The answer might be to purchase a computer, but you need to think very carefully about what you might want to use a computer for, how easy it is to use, and what support you will have in terms of help with programs or the machine itself, if you get stuck. Increasingly there are local classes being run for older or disabled people in the use of computers.

Chairs and wheelchairs

The last thing I want to do is to use a wheelchair, but I think I am going to have to consider it. Do I really have to?

If walking aids are seen by people with MS as the first visible stage of disability, then wheelchairs are often thought of as meaning 'the end of the road'. You may say, when you first learn that you have MS, 'I will never be seen in a wheelchair' or, even more dramatically, 'I would rather be dead than use a wheelchair'. To some, the wheelchair stands for 'being disabled' and, in a sense, for 'being useless'. It is no wonder that, for many people with MS, the day when they feel that they have to consider using a wheelchair is a big day in their lives. However, it is important to say that all people, with or without MS, have to adapt to declining mobility as they get older, and to using additional means of getting around. Although there are still major problems of access and, to a degree, still some social stigma attached to being in a wheelchair, the situation has dramatically changed in the last few years. This is not only because of social changes in relation to disabled people, e.g. through the Disability Discrimination Act and the focus on disabled people's rights, but also because of changes in wheelchair design, the use of wheelchairs for highly successful sports activities, and the advent of the electric scooter. In other words we are entering a new era, in which the use of wheelchairs as mobility aids will mean less dependence on others than it has in the past, and in which there is a new perspective on people with wheelchairs, backed up by legislation.

Although MS may speed up a little some of the things we have to manage as we get older, and our approach to them, the transition to life in a wheelchair is often not so bad. Actually considering the use of a wheelchair may be a relief – in the sense that it can help avoid some of the most awkward and exhausting struggles to get around in other ways, both for you or your partner or family members. In any case, you may only need it initially on an occasional basis.

When do you think that I should get a wheelchair?

The best approach to this issue is not so much thinking of walking (or struggling to walk) everywhere, and then making a complete change in one day to using a wheelchair all the time, but making a gradual transition, if you can, over weeks, months or years. When you find that:

- the effort, perhaps particularly outside the home, required to walk some distance is too much;
- walking aids tend to assist you less, and
- you are getting increasingly concerned about falling

then it will be worth considering using a wheelchair, at least for some activities. All but a few people with MS should be able to make a gradual transition to a wheelchair. This may overcome the 'all or nothing' approach, which many people with MS seem to fear. If it is outside the home that you need to use a wheelchair first, you could think of getting around in a combination of ways: using a wheelchair for some things and a walking aid for others. Where there are sufficient supports – perhaps around the home – you may be able to walk relatively unaided for a few steps. In this way, you can conserve your precious energy, still undertake some active exercise, and maybe actually increase the range of activities that you are able to do.

It is important that you obtain a good independent advice about the appropriate type and specification of wheelchair for your needs. An increasing number of companies are now producing wheelchairs of all kinds but it is best to ask someone who professionally assesses wheelchairs, usually an occupational therapist or a physiotherapist. The NHS also operates Wheelchair

Service Centres, where assessment is undertaken, and to which you should be referred for advice.

You might be able to get financial help via the mobility components of the Disability Living Allowance. Look in the *Disability Rights Handbook* (see Appendix 2), or telephone the Benefits Agency, the MS Society's Helpline, or your local DIAL (Disability Information and Advice Service). Appendix 1 has details of these.

Driving

What help is available for drivers?

There are a number of benefits for which you may be eligible. If you receive the higher rate mobility allowance, you will be allowed to claim exemption from vehicle excise duty (road tax) on one vehicle. This exemption is given on condition that the vehicle is used 'solely for the purposes of the disabled person', so care must be taken as to the use of the vehicle. Nevertheless, it is likely that some commonsense latitude will be given.

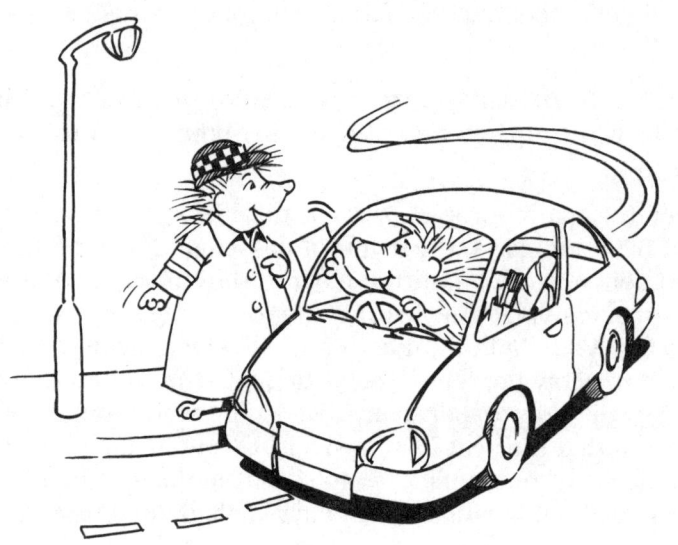

If you have the higher rate mobility allowance, you will be automatically eligible for the **Orange Badge** which gives parking privileges, and also for access to the Motability Scheme (see below). You will also get VAT exemption on adaptations to make your car suitable, as well as exemption on the repair, maintenance or replacement of these adaptations.

If you want an adapted car, the Department of Transport has set up a Mobility Advice and Vehicle Information Service (**MAVIS**) to help people choose an appropriate car for their needs,

For people with MS who are receiving a higher rate mobility component of the Disability Living Allowance (DLA), the **Motability Scheme** can offer a good approach to the purchase of a new car, good used car or an electric wheelchair, through hire purchase. Alternatively, you can hire a car through the same scheme.

If you decide to give up your car, consider getting an outdoor electric wheelchair or an electric scooter (sometimes called pavement vehicles) which, depending on the terrain near where you live, could be of great help in giving you more independence and ability to travel reasonable distances for shopping or leisure activities.

There are other forms of transport that you may find helpful, but these tend to vary according to which area you are living in. You can get in touch with your local authority for advice.

My wife has difficulty getting in and out of our car. I don't want to buy another one at present. What can I do to help her?

One of the major problems for a disabled person is swinging round from outside the car into a passenger, or a driver's seat, and of course getting out of the car in the same way. Depending on how much you want to spend, and exactly what your wife's needs are, you could think either of a swivel cushion placed on the seat to allow her legs to be swung into the car; or, more elaborately (and more expensively), replacing whole seats and their fittings so that the seat itself swivels; this will allow her to back on to the seat from outside, or to rise from the seat to a standing position without having to manoeuvre in and out of the car.

**I am concerned that my licence might be taken away if I
have MS. What's the position on this?**

You do have to notify the DVLA (Driver Vehicle and Licensing
Agency) that you have MS. You will receive a form PK1
(Application for Driving Licence/Notification of Driving Licence
Holder's State of Health) to complete and return. These forms
can be obtained at your local Post Office.

If you have been only recently diagnosed, you are unlikely to
lose your licence. The DVLA will consider the information that
you have given on the form and, if it believes that your driving
ability is not a hazard to other road users, it will normally issue a
three-year licence. Your situation will be reviewed at the end of
these three years. If you answer positively to any of the questions
concerning health problems on form PK1, then you should send a
covering letter explaining your situation, and why you believe
that you are fit to drive. Without such a letter or explanation, the
DVLA might withdraw your licence. It would also be worth
talking to your doctor – GP or neurologist – about your driving
ability. If they disagree with you about your capacity to drive, or
between themselves, or you yourself have concerns about your
driving ability, then you should arrange for an assessment at one
of the special driving and mobility assessment centres, which you
can find via the Department of Transport's Mobility Advice and
Vehicle Information Service (MAVIS) (see Appendix 1). There is a
charge for a driving assessment and this may vary depending on
the type of assessment required, so it is important to find out the
cost when you arrange it.

There is an appeals procedure if you do lose your licence, but it can
be lengthy and complex; you need to seek advice and consider the
likelihood of success, as well as the consequences of not succeeding.
It is worth talking to those, for example in the MS Society (see
Appendix 1), who will be able to offer both support and information.

There are some insurance companies who are now specializing
in insuring disabled drivers. A list is obtainable through RADAR
(*Mobility Fact Sheet No. 6*) which sets out these companies, and
broadly what they offer (see Appendix 2). It may be that you
could even lower your premium!

11
Speech and eating difficulties, problems with eyesight and hearing

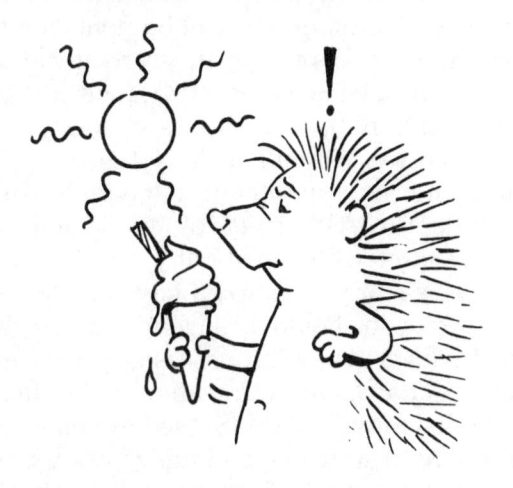

This chapter discusses problems you may get with speech, eating and swallowing. We then give some helpful hints for following a good diet. Some people experience problems with their eyesight or hearing. The final section discusses these.

Speech

Whilst difficulty with speech is perhaps one of the more obvious problems that you might face at some point, speech is only one of the ways in which we communicate – although it is a very important one – and thus it is crucial to consider speech in this context. Such things as facial expression, body movement and gesture are all linked with speech, in order to communicate our thoughts and needs. Nevertheless, it is speech itself which is often the focus of concern both for people with and without MS. As with other symptoms of MS, problems with speech can vary, particularly in the earlier stages of the disease.

As MS can potentially affect the control of most muscles, it is not surprising that it can affect those muscles which control voice production. Communication in general, and what others might think about how you communicate, worries many people with MS. Although the problem cannot currently be remedied by curing the neurological problem, appropriate advice, support and exercises can improve things considerably.

People say to me, 'Are you drunk?' I know that's what I sound like when my voice is bad, but how can I overcome this?

The first thing is to be aware of when your speech is unclear or slurred. Ask others sympathetically to accept that you have a problem. You can help by being much more deliberate in your speech; trying to pronounce your words much more precisely; slowing down your normal pace of speech, and giving yourself more time by pausing periodically, so that you can maintain a good rhythm, even if you speak much more slowly than you would normally.

You can also help yourself by learning to breathe in ways that assist the production of speech – indeed coordinated breathing in sequence with your speech is crucial. You may have to make a judgement about the length of your sentences and where you pause, so that you can try and maintain an effective, even if slightly slower, pace of speech.

If you can manage your level of fatigue well, and reduce or shorten the effects of exacerbations or attacks of MS, you may find that you have fewer problems with your speech.

Eating and swallowing

Will I develop problems eating or swallowing?

Most people with MS never experience major problems eating, chewing and swallowing, but it is difficult to indicate for certain who will and who will not develop these symptoms, for MS develops so variably. Many different muscles control the processes involved (similar to those involved in the process of speech); if MS has affected the relevant nerves controlling some or all of these muscles, then it is likely that at least some problems will become evident. Like other symptoms, these may be temporary or more permanent, depending on the degree and type of damage to the particular nervous tissue.

I have real problems swallowing solid food. What can I do about it?

If you do begin to have problems swallowing, then you ought first to seek the advice of your GP or neurologist, who may well refer you to a therapist for further advice and support. It is important to identify the nature of the problem, and to try various ways to help you eat and swallow more comfortably, such as:

- changing the type and preparation of your food – solid foods, particularly those which are only half chewed, are much more difficult to swallow than those which are softer, so you may need to consider chopping or blending food;

- changing the ways in which you eat and swallow – eating little and often may help;

- exercising to strengthen the relevant muscles as much as possible.

Why do I have the same problem swallowing liquids?

There may be particular difficulty experienced with some liquids, especially those which are less viscous and 'dense'. This is because the liquids pass through the mouth 'too fast' before the slower moving muscles have a chance to coordinate swallowing, so there is a risk of coughing and choking, as liquids might run into the airway to the lungs. Usually this problem is solved by thickening the liquids, so that they pass through the mouth more slowly and stand a far greater chance of being swallowed.

Diet and nutrition

Diet is the most obvious and easiest thing to change, and many people have focused on this issue. Essential fatty acids, which form part of the building blocks of the brain and nervous system tissue, are essential to the development and maintenance of the CNS. There are, of course, many kinds of 'fats'. Saturated fats are found in meat and dairy produce, and too much is not good for you; unsaturated and polyunsaturated fats, found in vegetable sources and from some of which the essential fatty acids are derived, are broadly good for you. About 60% of normal nervous system tissue is made up of these essential fatty acids. Some research has suggested that these were present in lower quantities in the CNS of people with MS than in that of people without the disease. The use of oil from the evening primrose plant, and some other oils, has become quite common amongst people with MS, for they do provide some of these missing constituents in a 'purer' form. It is not clear, however, whether taking large doses of such oils does return the levels of fatty acids to normal or, even if the levels are returned to 'normal', whether this will affect the course of MS, for the CNS damage has already been under way for some time.

If I decide to have additional essential fatty acids in my diet, what should I take?

Foods rich in essential fatty acids are those such as:

• sunflower and safflower seed oil

• evening primrose oil

- offal such as liver; kidney, brains, sweetbread
- lean meat
- green vegetables
- fish and seafood
- fish liver oils
- linseeds.

The oil of the evening primrose plant has become a very popular dietary supplement for people with MS, because it is unique and contains large quantities of a substance called gamma-linoleic acid, a more complex form of linoleic acid which is converted into further important fatty acids by the body. Some other rarer oils may also contain good quantities of gamma-linoleic acid.

What about more general diets and MS? You talked earlier about the balance between saturated, and poly- or non-saturated fats. If I reduced my intake of saturated fats, would that make any difference to my MS?

People argue about whether changes in your saturated fat intake will make any difference to your MS. If, in general, essential fatty acids are 'good', then you could increase your intake of these as we have noted, and/or reduce your intake of the 'bad' saturated fats. Of course, there are general health grounds for suggesting that you should lower your intake of saturated fats, but some people who have devised low saturated fat diets for their MS claim that such diets may be far more beneficial for their MS.

I have heard of things called 'exclusion diets' for MS. Are they likely to help?

Cutting out saturated fats is an exclusion diet, but there are other diets that cut out many more specific substances. MS symptoms are considered by some people to be an allergic reaction to certain foods or drinks, and this view has led to other exclusion diets. One such diet is the gluten-free diet, where it is argued that gluten has produced damage in the digestive and elimination system and has made the MS worse. Thus by eliminating gluten it is hoped that damage to the intestine can be prevented. Such diets were developed from those for people with coeliac disease who cannot absorb fats when gluten is present from cereal grains. At one stage these diets gained considerable popularity, but the burden placed on people with MS to stick to a very rigid gluten-free diet, together with disappointing results for many people and a lack of scientific support, has led to their decline.

The relative success claimed for very different diets in particular individuals suggests not so much that these diets are improving MS, but that concomitant problems are possibly being helped in some way by the diets. Of course, if your general health is better, you will feel better, and certain (but not all) symptoms of your MS might be a little improved. The key issue is balancing whatever benefits that you may be gaining against the costs, time and resources that you have to devote to maintaining what can be a formidable dietary regimen.

If you feel that MS will not necessarily be affected by dietary change, what would you suggest I do in relation to eating and drinking?

There are certain general dietary principles now widely accepted for general health which, on those grounds alone, should be considered by people with MS. These include:

- very little intake of saturated fat (with very limited dairy produce, and generally only certain specific cuts of meat, liver for example);

- plenty of fish;

- a plentiful intake of vegetables and salads – either raw or as lightly cooked as possible;

- pulses;

- plenty of fresh fruit;

- a good intake of most nuts, seeds and seed oils (but excluding those containing saturated oils and certain nuts containing saturated fats, such as brazil nuts);

- as little as possible refined carbohydrates, sugar, processed or packaged foods;

- cutting down on alcohol consumption, and

- cutting out smoking.

In addition, if you want to supplement this diet with liver and evening primrose oil, for example, it will not do you any harm, as long as you don't feel these supplements are adding greatly to your budget.

What about vitamin and mineral supplements? I am sure that I have read that people with MS have deficiencies in some key vitamins and minerals. Wouldn't it be good to take those?

Most of the diets used by people with MS appear to be also supplemented by various vitamins and minerals. The value of these for MS itself is unclear, although there is a mountain of popular information suggesting that most vitamins and minerals in our bodies need supplementing. However, there is little scientific evidence that the average healthy adult with a reasonably balanced diet needs any significant vitamin or mineral supplements. The key questions for people with MS are:

- How much has your general health been compromised and do you need supplementation for this?

- Will additional vitamins and minerals help your MS?

As far as general health is concerned, it is clearly important that people with MS receive a balanced intake of vitamins and minerals appropriate to their age, gender and situation. This can best be undertaken through a balanced diet, of the general kind we have mentioned above. Supplementation should only be necessary where, for various reasons, it is not possible to follow such a diet. There is little scientific evidence that supplementing beyond this general level will produce significant health benefits, although many popular books appear to suggest so. As for the specific value of such supplements for the MS itself, again there is little evidence of major value, except where there are scientifically established deficiencies – and this is a relatively unusual situation.

As to vitamins and minerals, there is no scientific evidence that serious deficiencies can damage the nervous system as evident in MS. You should be very careful with vitamin supplements, especially megadoses. Vitamins A and D, in particular, are toxic in high doses; vitamin B6 can produce symptoms in the peripheral nervous system at high doses, and vitamin C in very high doses can produce stomach problems and kidney stones. Overall, evidence suggests that, apart from taking care that you have a normal balanced intake of vitamins, there is little to be gained from major supplementation of vitamins in your diet. A similar position seems to apply to mineral supplementation.

Eyesight and hearing

My eyesight is getting worse, and is very bad when my MS is bad. Why is this?

There may be a number of possibilities here. You are probably experiencing the periodic symptoms of what is called *optic neuritis*. This is a name for inflammation of and subsequent damage to the optic nerve at the back of the eye, when your symptoms may occur. Problems with eyesight (particularly if they are transient at first, such as double vision) are often con-sidered one of the first likely signs of MS, particularly if they are associated with a damaged optic nerve on clinical examination. Vision problems as a result of optic neuritis can indeed occur many years before other symptoms of the disease are seen.

Although it is unusual for someone with MS to lose their sight completely (although this can occasionally happen temporarily), many people have episodes during which their sight will become worse. Only one, or both eyes may be affected, and your sight may be disturbed in various ways, including:

- double vision (*diplopia*);

- a blank field or spot in the middle of your vision (*scotoma*);

- loss of peripheral vision;

- blurring of vision;

- problems with colour vision or certain contrasts, such as an unusual balance between light and shade in the visual field;

- pain with inflammation of the optic nerve;

- visual disturbance after exercise (*Uthoff's phenomenon*);

- *nystagmus* – a rapid flickering of one or both eyes, perhaps more evident to others, which is painless.

On occasions high-dose corticosteroids (such as methyl-prednisolone or dexamethasone) have helped some visual problems that are symptoms of MS and that may be worse during MS 'attacks' but, like other powerful drugs, they may have side effects. Clonazepam (Rivotril) can sometimes help nystagmus. However, your doctor will need to advise you about the role of these or other drugs, in assisting any visual problems that you may have.

Just a final point here. Of course eyesight problems can occur for many other reasons than MS – people may have short or long sight or other visual problems, for which glasses or contact lenses will be useful and, as they age, some of these problems will become more evident to people with MS. Be sure to have these problems, and those specifically caused by the MS itself, checked out.

I think my hearing is affected as I can't hear so well now. Is this the MS?

The answer is almost certainly no. MS is not known to cause significant symptoms in hearing (although there can always be the occasional exception), even if a test called an 'auditory evoked response' (see Chapter 4) reveals some damage to the relevant nerves. Very, very occasionally some hearing loss may occur temporarily as a result of the MS but, if your hearing loss is gradual or persistent, it needs investigating for other causes.

12
Living with MS

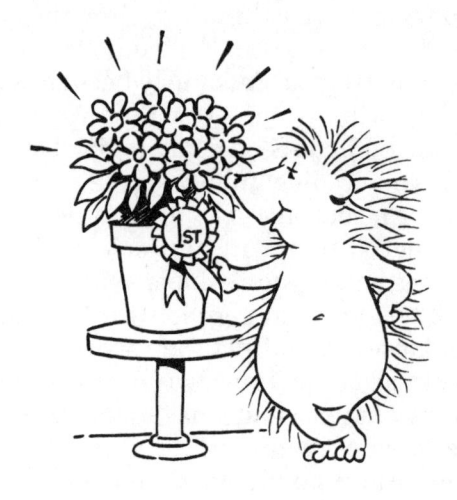

Many of the key issues affecting people with MS and their families concern practical problems of managing employment, housing, insurance and other financial problems, leisure and holidays, dealing with social services, as well as investigating possibilities for respite and long-term care in MS.

Employment and MS

Can I do my job now that I have been diagnosed with MS?

Intrinsically there is no reason why, once you have been diagnosed with MS, you should not be able to do your job. The key

131

issues are, as they were before, your ability and capacity to do your job; your confidence in them, and the organization, support and facilities that your employer makes available.

Overall, however, MS is such a variable condition that it is really not possible to say whether your symptoms will make it difficult for you to do your job. Some people never experience any significant symptoms during their working life, as they have a mild form of MS. For other people it may depend not only on the type of symptoms that arise, but how often they occur, and the particular type of work involved. For example, a job that involves very close attention to visual detail may become a problem if you have difficulties with your eyesight. Work that involves memorizing facts and figures on a day-to-day basis may be made more difficult if you are beginning to have more problems with your memory. Work that involves a great deal of walking and lifting may become difficult if you have problems with your mobility. Although some people have symptoms that progress quite quickly, the majority of people with MS will have specific symptoms or relapses that affect their work for no more than a few days or weeks at a time. However, you may have to be careful about the effects of fatigue, and you should try and pace yourself within your work to deal with this.

Two other important points need to be made here. First it is vital to consider your own feelings about your ability to do your work. Some people with MS seem to doubt their own abilities unnecessarily, often as soon as the diagnosis is made. The second point is just as important: whether you can do a job depends on the facilities, circumstances and support you receive from your employer, as much as it does on your abilities. Your employer is legally bound under certain categories of the Disability Discrimination Act 1995 to give you certain kinds of support.

Now that I have been diagnosed with MS, do I have to tell my employer?

The formal position is that you are not obliged to tell your existing employer anything about your personal circumstances, except where they affect your ability to perform your duties, or where you have a contract that specifically requires you to do so. Your ability to perform your duties is an issue for you to determine, in consultation with your doctor. You need only to inform your employer if you feel that you are unable to cope with your contractual obligations (those set out in your contract of employment) or the duties that you have taken on in practice (which may be quite different from your contract). In either case, you will need to explain your circumstances when it is clear that your ability to do your job safely will be affected.

Employment contracts that require disclosure of health circumstances are rare, and are very individual in nature. In some cases there may be clear health and safety reasons for including this as a condition of employment (such as operating machinery or vehicles), but this is not necessarily so. For most people, it is not so much the ability to perform at work which presents difficulties as the uncertainty of future circumstances and the need for irregular absences from work. Although you may not need to disclose MS, it is advisable to inform your employer if you need time off from work for medical reasons in advance, rather than waiting for absences to be noticed.

Despite the formal situation, however, some people find that keeping their MS a secret from their employer is very difficult and stressful. It may also mean that, through circumstances not of your choosing, your employer gets to hear of your MS accidentally, and you may not be able to discuss your situation as easily as you would like if this happens. You may also have underestimated the degree of support and understanding that you might receive if you tell your employer. Many of the larger employers are now getting used to dealing sympathetically and well with people with MS, although some smaller employers are still less aware of MS and may be less sympathetic to your situation. The publicity attached to the implementation of the Disability Discrimination Act 1995 should help to inform more employers, and the MS Society is taking considerable steps to provide this information to them.

I understand that the provisions of the Disability Discrimination Act 1995 apply to many aspects of employment for people with disabilities. How might it affect someone with MS?

The provisions of the Disability Discrimination Act 1995 are in principle very substantial, and apply to many aspects of employment. However, the exact implications of many of the provisions have not yet been legally tested, so it will only become clear over the next few years how precisely the Act will apply. It is important to remember that the Act applies to organizations and companies with over 15 employees, although those with under this number are expected to abide by the spirit of the provisions.

Broadly, the position under the Act is that unlawful discrimination in employment occurs in the following circumstances:

• when a disabled person is treated less favourably than someone else;

• this treatment is given for a reason relating to that person's disability;

• the reason does not apply to the other person, and

• the treatment cannot be justified.

Such discrimination must not occur in the recruitment and retention of employees; promotion and transfers; training and development, and the dismissal process. In addition employers must make reasonable changes to their premises or employment arrangements if these substantially disadvantage a disabled employee, or prospective employee, compared to a non-disabled person.

Can I be sacked because I have MS? What legal protection is there for people in my position?

Legally, you cannot be sacked for having a diagnosis of MS unless this is a condition written into your contract of employment (which is highly unlikely). You can be sacked for failing to perform your duties, in which case the reason for failing to perform your duties is not relevant. Therefore, if you are working and able to continue working on the same basis that you did before your diagnosis, you cannot be legally sacked because of the symptoms of MS.

If you are unable to work, you are protected by limited legislation that provides sickness pay according to the terms of your contract (employer's sick pay) and this is usually limited to a certain number of days per year or a fixed term. Beyond that is government sickness pay (statutory sick pay) which is also limited. Many smaller companies do not operate a sick pay scheme of course. If you have either health insurance or pension arrangements, privately or through employment, they are likely to exceed sick pay in the event that you are no longer able to work.

Apart from legal protection, your employer may be willing to negotiate a change in your terms of employment, such as a change in duties or a change in working patterns (part-time or non-shift work) and, under the Disability Discrimination Act (see above), they may be under a legal obligation to do so. Additionally it is in your employer's interest to keep experienced or trained staff.

I am finding it rather difficult to find a job that I can do now that my MS has become more severe.

Job Centre employment service staff should provide services for all disabled people to help you find a job. If your situation is more complex because of your disability, you may be referred to a Disability Employment Advisor (DEA) in the Placement, Assessment and Counselling Team (PACT). In addition to giving advice, DEAs can try and help you into a job using various schemes available through government support.

If I apply for a new job, am I obliged to tell my prospective employers about my MS?

If you are not asked, and a medical examination is not required, then the answer is no. However, in most circumstances, it will be almost impossible not to inform your prospective employers about your condition; it would be wrong to deceive them if asked, or if a medical examination is undertaken. Deception itself about your situation could result in serious consequences. It is important to note that your diagnosis itself is, under current legislation, insufficient grounds not to employ you, so long as you are fit and able to work. These points should be stressed when the issue arises, although as we have already pointed out, it is crucial that your employer is aware of supportive information about MS from other sources such as the MS Society.

Should I tell my colleagues about my MS?

There is no easy answer to your question – it is entirely up to you how to manage your relationships with your colleagues at work. However, given the way that news gets around, it is unlikely that you will be able to tell one colleague without others becoming aware of your situation quite quickly. Despite your wishes, sometimes it can even happen that information from outside your work situation alerts colleagues about your MS unintentionally, for example an inadvertent message from a family member to a colleague about an absence from work. Thus it is probably wise to work out ways in which to tell your colleagues in a planned process.

Finances

This section deals with some very complicated issues. This is not only because people's own circumstances are all different, but because the rules and regulations governing eligibility to benefits, pensions and so on are themselves complex, and moreover appear to change very frequently. The government is currently considering major changes to legislation concerning state benefits for disabled people. It is very important that, in addition to taking note of the points we make below, you consult other sources of information. Choices that you may make about continuing or leaving work, or about benefits or pensions, may have long-lasting consequences, so it is important to think them through carefully, after seeking impartial advice.

Sources of information include:

- *Disability rights handbook*, published by the Disability Alliance (see Appendix 2)

- the Benefits Agency

- Citizens' Advice Bureaux

- your local authority and the MS Society's Welfare Rights Advisor

- Post Offices

- Employment Service Offices.

Financial help for drivers is discussed in Chapter 10 under *Driving*.

I have MS. Am I entitled to any help while I am still working?

There are a number of possible sources of support for you if you are still working and have MS.

- As we have noted above, under the Disability Discrimination Act there are certain obligations laid on many employers to provide additional facilities, adaptations and changes in working practice so as not to discriminate against people with disabilities. What these sources of support might be in your case would depend on more information about your situation and that of your employer.

- If you are working at least 16 hours each week and have a child, you may be eligible for Family Credit; or, if you are working 16 hours a week and also already getting a 'qualifying incapacity or disability benefit', you may be eligible for the Disability Working Allowance. Depending on the level of your income you might also be eligible for Housing Benefit, and a number of other benefits.

- If you require specialized equipment of any kind which is generally helpful and supportive, such as a stairlift, but it is not available to you through NHS or Social Service sources, you may find that charitable, professional or trade union funds could help (see below).

I have had increasing problems of sickness owing to MS over the last few months, and thus have had to take a lot of time off work. What benefits might I be eligible for?

If you remain off work sick, you can apply for Income Support (which is a non-contributory means-tested benefit). If you are considered medically incapable of work, you may be eligible for Incapacity Benefit and for Disability Living Allowance. The Citizens Advice Bureau can tell you whether you are eligible for these benefits. If you continue working you may be eligible for the Disability Working Allowance, but taking this allowance may have consequences for other benefits; again, you need to seek advice from an impartial source about your options.

If I decide to stop working completely, what are likely to be the financial consequences, and what benefits will I get?

The answer to your question is that it depends very much on your personal circumstances, the extent of your disability from MS, the nature of your occupation and any health insurance and/or early retirement pensions provision, amongst other factors. This is why you need careful and detailed impartial advice from someone who is able to go through all the aspects of your situation, and point out both the short- and long-term financial consequences of any decision you make.

Are there any other benefits that I might be able to obtain?

Yes, you could seek help for a particular piece of equipment or a particular service you need. Funds are often held by trade unions, professional organizations or charitable bodies for such purposes, and these may be given for holidays. Often there is a question of eligibility, but of a different kind than that for the Benefits Agency. You may have to be a current or former member of the organization concerned, or have some other characteristic which gives you entitlement – such as living in a particular area. The problem is often finding out which organizations you can apply to, for many local charities are small and are not widely advertised. However, there is a *Charities digest* (your local library should have a copy) which lists many, although not all, sources of funds. Your local library, or the Citizen's Advice Bureau, may be able to give you some sources as well. There is also another directory called *A guide to grants for individuals in need* which contains a relatively comprehensive list of charities who provide support for individuals with certain eligibility criteria (see Appendix 2). The MS Society can help here too.

What is the Disability Living Allowance and who can claim it?

This is an allowance that has replaced the Attendance Allowance for people aged under 65. It is paid to people who require personal care or supervision in the daytime or at night and/or to people who have mobility problems. There are three levels of funding for the care component and two levels of funding for the mobility component, and the care and mobility components are assessed separately. Forms can be obtained from the Benefits Agency. A wide range of people may be eligible for one or other component of this allowance, but it is important to seek the support of your GP or other health professional for your application, as their comments on your claim may be vital for its success.

Will I be able to claim Severe Disablement Allowance?

If you do not have a sufficiently complete National Insurance Contribution record to claim Incapacity Benefit, and on medical examination are able to meet an 80% test of disablement, you would be eligible for this benefit. A medical examiner is appointed by the Department of Social Security to assess you. This allowance counts as income for the calculation of all other benefits except Attendance Allowance and Disability Living Allowance.

Insurance

Do I have to tell my insurance company that I have MS?

In the case of health insurance, life assurance or endowment policies associated with a mortgage, yes you do. Such information may also be required for car insurance purposes in order to ensure that any future claim you make will not be denied, on the grounds that you had not told the company about MS. As you will probably be aware, insurance application forms generally have a 'catch-all' request that you provide 'any information that you feel may be relevant', or a similar wording. What this means is that, if you have failed to provide information that the insurance company – not just yourself – feels is relevant to a claim that you may make at a later date, then the claim could be invalidated and it will not be met. Thus in this case the burden is on you, as the insured or the applicant, to disclose information relevant to any future claim, and ensure that the full facts are given when the insurance is first taken out.

For existing policies, you are obliged to give all details of any changes in your circumstances, whenever your insurance is renewed. However, so long as the changes in circumstances (e.g. a diagnosis of MS) occurred after you took out the policy, there should – in principle – be no substantial change in the terms of your insurance, although the company may make enquiries as to whether in fact you did know about the MS when taking out that insurance.

Almost all health insurance policies carry exclusions for 'pre-existing conditions' which is taken to mean any condition of which there was significant evidence before insurance commenced. In the case of a condition such as MS, this would include any tests or examinations that you have had that related to MS, including all those that you underwent before diagnosis. It is wise to be as accurate and as detailed as possible to give as few grounds as you can for exclusion at a later date as possible. It is worth noting that few insurance companies will refuse to insure you, although most will charge higher premiums when there is a reasonable cause to expect a higher risk of claims.

Do be careful to read the terms of any attractive policy which guarantees acceptance and has fixed premiums. The maximum payout and range of exclusions may seriously limit the value of the cover, and a 'no questions asked, no medicals' policy can still exclude claims where the insured failed to provide information when the cover was taken out.

Do mortgage lenders and insurance companies discriminate against people who have MS?

It is not possible to give an across-the-board answer to you. Many factors are taken into account when you ask for a mortgage, including your savings, your income and the security of your employment, and of course how much you may wish to borrow. However, the key factor will be the company's estimation of how likely you will be able to continue paying for your mortgage until its term is complete. In this respect, different companies may take a different view of the future, partly depending on whether they feel you will be able to keep in employment for the term of the mortgage. Some may take a more pessimistic view than others of the progress and effects of your MS, so it is important that you shop around, as with other major financial transactions that you may make.

Although insurance companies can, and sometimes do refuse to insure people with conditions like MS, their usual response is to load the premiums according to the risks they estimate of you making a claim. Thus you may find quite big differences between insurance companies in the way they respond to information about MS. A 'niche' insurance market has begun to specialize in people with disabilities and certain kinds of medical condition, and there are now life policies, particularly for older people over 50, which guarantee acceptance and pay out fixed sums after two years without a medical examination or other questions asked, although see the points made in the previous question about such policies. In all cases you need to seek impartial advice, to shop around, and to consider very carefully any conditions or exclusions to policies – in short you must read the small print!

Health care finance

Am I entitled to free prescriptions?

Unfortunately you are not entitled to free prescriptions just because you have MS – it is not yet included as one of the relatively few diseases or conditions for which free prescriptions are available. However, prescriptions are free if you are aged under 16 or in full-time education and aged under 19; if you are aged over 60; or if you are either pregnant, or have had a baby within the last 12 months. In these cases you need only to sign the appropriate section of the prescription form. Prescriptions are also free when you are receiving many forms of state benefit and this may also apply to your partner and dependent children.

If you or your partner are on state benefits (specifically Income Support, Jobseeker's Allowance, Family Credit, or Disability Working Allowance), you can also claim free prescriptions. Some prescriptions are also free for people receiving hospital care or diagnosed with very specific medical conditions not including MS itself, but including some of its possible complications such as genitourinary infections. There are also a number of other specific circumstances in which free prescriptions may be available, and these need to be checked out with your local Social Security Office.

In some of these circumstances you will require a completed HC1, HC2 or HC3 form and certificate number. You can obtain the form from a Social Security office, NHS hospital, dentist or doctor.

Even if you are not entitled to free prescriptions, you can save money if you need more than five items in 4 months or more than 14 items in 12 months by using a pre-payment certificate. You will need to get an application form FP95 from a Post Office or pharmacy.

Can I also claim for eye and dental care costs?

In addition to free prescriptions, most of the categories of entitlement listed above also entitle you to NHS (not private) dental care, eye tests and glasses or contact lenses. Necessary costs of travel to hospital for NHS treatment include the cost of travel for a partner or helper if you are unable to travel alone.

Given the high costs of prescription, eye care and dental treatment, it is well worth exercising your claim to whatever qualifying benefits you are entitled to, in order then to have these free treatments, even if you feel the qualifying benefit itself is of relatively little value to you.

Care in the community

I am going to have a 'needs assessment'. What will this involve?

A needs assessment is organized by Social Services when they think that someone may need community services. The assessment is usually carried out either by a social worker or an occupational therapist; you will have to complete a questionnaire. The views of the GP will be taken into account – and thus it will be important to discuss your situation with your GP before the assessment, so that you are clear as to his or her position on your needs. The views of other professional staff who have had contact with you, or who have assessed you for other purposes, may also be considered in the needs assessment. If you have someone caring for you, they may also be involved in the assessment – but not necessarily so, for the assessment is actually only of your own needs, not the needs of any carer.

After the needs assessment has been carried out, Social Services should discuss with you what services are available to meet your needs. Assuming that the Social Services assessment indicates that your needs do require their support, then they should also appoint a 'care manager' to manage a 'care plan' –

which will state the nature, type and frequency of community services you may receive.

What role will a 'care manager' take in my life?

A 'care manager' is the person (usually a social worker) who manages your care plan following your needs assessment. You should be provided with a copy of the needs assessment and the care plan. The care manager should monitor the care plan and make appropriate changes to it as your situation changes. The care manager is important as the main line of communication to the Social Services Department, and the main means through whom any problems can be remedied or resolved. A good care manager will be supportive and helpful.

What kinds of services might be available following a needs assessment and care plan?

In principle many services can be provided through a care plan following a needs assessment. However, financial constraints and the differential availability of services locally may mean that relatively few are available for any one person. The list in the box opposite shows (again in principle!) the kinds of services which *might* be made available through a care plan, or associated with it, depending on the results of the needs assessment, local resources available, and the organization of health, social service and voluntary sector cooperation.

I care for my wife. Could I be assessed for my needs?

If you are the main carer of a person with MS, and you share the house with that person, or you look after him or her on a regular and substantial basis, then you can request your own needs assessment. This is not a check as to whether you are 'good' at caring, it is to check whether you are getting the support you need to carry on caring if you want to.

Carers' needs assessments are carried out by Social Services Departments under the arrangements in the Carers (Recognition

Services available in your home

- adaptations of various kinds
- alarm systems
- various benefits
- equipment
- help from Good Neighbour or Care Attendant schemes
- home helps or carers
- home visits from various professionals
- homemaker schemes (someone to look after your home if your carer temporarily cannot)
- home library service
- laundry service
- meals on wheels
- odd job schemes (practical help for odd jobs in the home)
- recreational facilities (TV and radio)
- sitting in or sleeping in services (allowing a carer a day or night away)
- social work support
- telephone services.

Services available outside the home

- day centres
- day hospital care
- education work centres
- holiday/short-term care
- medical escort service (to get to hospital)
- respite or short-stay care.

Medical services

- occupational therapy
- physiotherapy
- speech and language therapy
- general rehabilitation.

and Services) Act (1995). Such a needs assessment can be considered only in conjunction with a needs assessment of your wife. If your wife has been assessed previously, or if her circumstances have changed, you may have to ask for her to be assessed again.

Unfortunately, even if your needs are assessed, Social Services are not under any legal obligation to provide you with help. However, if you have an assessment, it may put you in a stronger position to argue for more support or, for example, respite care. You need to remember that formally Social Services are technically responsible for the care of your wife. Any support that you give her is up to you, and so they must take account of the needs of your wife, without taking your care for granted.

The Carers National Association has a helpline which provides advice on carers' needs assessments. It publishes helpful booklets on caring aspects (see Appendix 1 and 2 for details).

Home adaptations

We have got to the point where my wife with MS cannot really get up the stairs any more. What are our options on staying in the house or should we move?

The choices will depend on what you both wish to do, your income, how easy the home is to adapt, and what kinds of services are available from the local Social Services and Housing Departments.

If you are happy with your current home in all respects apart from the stairs, then you could consider having a stair lift installed. You could pay for this yourself or you can apply to the Social Services Department to see if you meet their eligibility criteria for financial support. You may be able to obtain a Disabled Facilities Grant which is available for adapting a property for the needs of a disabled person. There is a range of eligibility criteria as with other benefits. Some of the grants are mandatory for specific purposes, in particular for access and making the dwelling safe amongst other things, and awards are discretionary in that they can be made available depending on local policies and the case concerned.

Another possibility would be to move downstairs, but this could lead to a major change in your family relationships. So other housing might be better for you and this will depend on finance, and on whether you own or rent your current home. Even if you do own your own home, if you are thinking seriously about moving, you could discuss the situation with the Housing Department of your local authority, as well as explore other options: for example, housing associations operating locally may have a special interest or concern for people with disabilities.

Respite and residential care

Sometimes a temporary and occasional break may be needed by the carer, and later a longer term and more permanent care outside the home may have to be arranged for the person with MS. Such decisions are always difficult because almost always they involve a separation from partners or other family members, and this adds to the anxieties and concerns of all parties to the discussions.

I look after my husband and have been told that I can have respite care. What is it exactly?

Respite care is the general name given to any facilities or resources which allows those who are involved in caring for people with significant caring needs, to have a break from their caring tasks. Such a break may take many forms. The Carers National Association has published a sensitive and helpful book-let called *Taking a break* (details in Appendix 2) which discusses the kinds of alternatives likely to be available, and also considers the hopes, fears and anxieties that may be associated with respite care. It also has examples of how respite care has worked for a number of people in different situations.

If you just need a few hours break, an organization called Crossroads Caring for Carers (see Appendix 1) can help here. Your Social Services Department may run Day Centres; others are run by the Women's Royal Voluntary Service or the Red Cross, or residential nursing homes.

Contact your Social Services Department also if you feel that you need a longer break. Again, local nursing or residential homes could meet your needs. Hospital care may be feasible for a very seriously disabled person. Unfortunately very few places as yet take couples when one partner has MS.

If the break is difficult financially, the local authority will assess your husband's ability to pay (not yours). The Citizen's Advice Bureau can give you advice about the costs involved.

You may like to talk things over with your GP, community nurse or the welfare officer of your local MS Society because any decision will be difficult. If you feel guilty about taking a break, remember that your well-being is crucial in the longer term to enable you to look after your husband.

Leisure and holidays

Since I have been diagnosed with MS, I've given up many interests that I had before, and this seems to make me even more preoccupied with the MS itself. My doctor and many of my friends urge me to take up the interests again. What do you think?

Yes, you should. Although MS itself may cause some problems from time to time, and interrupts your life more than you might like, it is important to keep your interests going as much as you can, not least because many of your interests will have given you a great deal of enjoyment in the past and no doubt will do so again. They will also enable you to keep in touch with old friends, and make new ones. Hobbies may help you to put MS far more in perspective.

I am worried about doing active things like sports or gardening, because the MS is beginning to affect my mobility. Will they harm me?

On the contrary, you should try keep as active as possible – especially if your mobility is affected. It is even more important that you try and exercise regularly to try and keep your muscles and joints working as well as you can. It is not so much what you do, but how you do it. Although not everyone will be able to do very vigorous exercise, activities like swimming and gardening are possible for many. For gardening, try raised beds or containers, both of which are easier to manage from a wheelchair. There is also a large range of tools for the handicapped gardener.

Information on local facilities for sport can be sought from The British Sports Association for the Disabled (see Appendix 1).

Information services on gardening include:

- DIAL (Disablement Information Advice Lines);
- the Disabled Living Foundation;
- Gardening for the Disabled Trust, and
- Horticultural Therapy.

There is also a book called *Grow it yourself: gardening with a physical disability*. See Appendices 1 and 2 for information on all these organizations and publications.

If you do have concerns about being active, or about undertaking a particular sport, do consult your doctor and/or a physiotherapist.

My husband and I like going out to places like the theatre and cinema or stately homes and gardens, but my MS has reduced my mobility, and I have to use a wheelchair on some occasions. We have found before that wheelchair access is often difficult, and sometimes impossible. What should we do?

Many managers of public places like these have generally been slow to understand and provide for the needs of people with disabilities until recently. Whilst many venues are more prepared for people with disabilities, it is still a good idea to contact the management before you go, to explain your situation and what you will need. In theatres, some positions for wheelchairs can be better than others and certain performances (for example, matinées) are less crowded than others.

Try the organizations below for information about your favourite places:

- London has an information service called Artsline.

- DIAL, RADAR (the Royal Association for Disability and Rehabilitation), local disability groups or your local MS Society, or your local authority information service may give advice on similar services in your area.

Publications that include a wealth of information are:

- *The National Trust handbook*

- *Places that care*

- *The National Gardens Scheme handbook*

- *Historic houses, castles and gardens.*

See Appendices 1 and 2 for more details. Some of your experiences may provoke you into joining one of the many local groups campaigning for better local access to public buildings and places!

We have found holidays increasingly difficult with my husband having MS, and we have not had a real holiday for a long time. Are there special sources of help or advice you could suggest?

All holidays require planning, and those which are organized for people with MS with mobility or other everyday problems, and often their families as well, require special consideration. It is perhaps almost too easy to 'give up' on holidays, not only perhaps for financial or related reasons, but also because travelling to unfamiliar places with people unfamiliar with the problems that MS might bring, can be very worrying. However, there are a number of sources of advice and support which can help you plan and enjoy a well deserved holiday.

The first thing to do is to decide in general terms what sort of holiday you would like, and particularly how far you would like to travel. You also need to think about how much care and attention you and your husband will need, to make your holiday enjoyable. Then you need to talk your ideas over with someone or some organization who knows what is available, its cost and so on. Officers as well as individual members of your local branch of the MS Society and nationally may have helpful information. Locally some branches of the MS Society organize holidays for their members with special needs.

Many holiday areas, and resorts now produce relatively detailed information – through information and/or tourist offices and the Internet – for people with special needs, on the accessibility of accommodation, and other facilities. Many Social Service Departments may also help. Some travel agents or coach operators offer special holidays for people with mobility problems – it is worth checking locally to see whether there are any in your area.

Two other national organizations provide information and advice for people with special needs of many kinds and their carers: the Holiday Care Service which advises on particular places for holidays, as well as on issues of transport, insurance and financial sources for funding a holiday; and RADAR (the Royal Association for Disability and Rehabilitation) who produces good information in guides, both on holidays in Britain and abroad (see Appendix 1 for details). The Holiday Care Service also has a service called Holiday Helpers which links specially selected volunteers with people like your wife.

Another organization called the Winged Fellowship Trust (see Appendix 1) may be very useful for people with MS and their families. It is a charity whose aim is to provide holidays for people with disabilities. It has a number of purpose-built or adapted holiday homes which can cater for people with severe mobility problems, and it recruits young volunteers to help look after the holidaymakers and ensure, as far as possible, that they have a good holiday.

If you go abroad, you should be sure to arrange adequate insurance cover, and tell your insurance company that you have MS to avoid any complications. Medical attention is free throughout the European Union as long as you have completed Form E111 (available from the Post Office) and take it with you when you go. Also, don't forget to take your medicines with you because some drugs may not be available abroad, or available only through specialists.

13
Sexual relationships

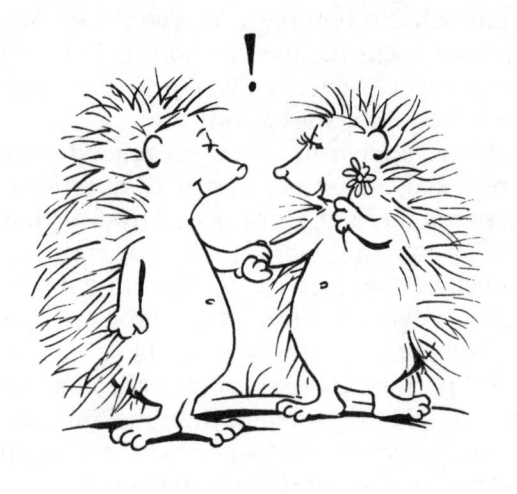

Many people are diagnosed with MS at a time when they are, or may be about to become sexually active, in their relationships. The issues associated with how best to manage sexual activity and MS has in the past often proved difficult to discuss with others. In this chapter, we address some of the common worries that men and women with MS, and their partners, may have.

As a relatively young man with MS, I am sure that I am having some sexual problems that I reckon are due to the MS. Do you think that's likely? Do other men with MS have sexual problems?

Of course sexual problems can take many forms, and almost all of them may affect people other than those with MS. As you may be aware, it is quite difficult to obtain accurate statistics about

153

the relative sexual problems of people with and without MS. Nevertheless, it does appear that sexual problems of several kinds do seem to be more likely amongst men with MS. Studies have shown that over 70% of men under 50 with mild MS have experienced problems in their sexual abilities compared to 20% in non-MS people; 80% found their erectile capacity and ejaculation diminished. There was a lower frequency of sexual intercourse in the great majority of men with MS, and their interest in or satisfaction with intercourse was also lower. Many men with MS have reported orgasmic dysfunction – often associated with premature or retarded ejaculation – problems with fatigue, as well as lower levels of masturbation.

Sexual problems appear to be closely related to problems with bladder or bowel dysfunction, and with spasticity in the legs. However, there are three kinds of sexual dysfunctions often associated with MS. Some problems are directly related to changes in the nerve pathways damaged by the MS – and this is often called **primary sexual dysfunction**. Other problems caused by MS that affect other parts of the body, or body systems, indirectly affecting sexual performance, are often called **secondary sexual dysfunction**. Yet other problems may be related to personal, social or cultural issues which make sexual activity more difficult – often called **tertiary sexual dysfunction**.

It is probable that all three dysfunctions can occur, either at the same time, or at different times, as well as influencing each other. For example, fears about future sexual performance (a tertiary dysfunction), partly derived from occasional or frequent erectile difficulties (often a primary dysfunction), may create further difficulties, compounded by mobility problems or fatigue (secondary dysfunctions). Disentangling the relationship between all these factors requires careful analysis and then management.

With my MS I'm really having a difficulty 'performing' sexually. Most the time I can't get an erection. What's the problem?

At a 'mechanical' level erections may not occur either because of problems in the blood supply to the penis, or problems in the control of erections and ejaculation by the nervous system, and this is much more likely in MS.

Managing erectile problems in principle mean focusing on three sets of possible problems: those in the nervous system; those associated with the blood supply system, and those arising from psychological and related issues. At present there are no means of restoring already damaged nervous system pathways, so the help is most effectively given through stimulation of the blood supply and resolving psychological problems.

You have talked about how MS might affect men's sexual lives; how about those of women?

If the study of men's sexual problems in MS has been neglected, the study of women's sexual problems has been even more so. In part this has been because mainstream medicine has marginalized women's sexual problems and traditionally the major emphasis of treatment has been on men's sexual performance. However, the situation is getting better with changing social values and with women themselves becoming more vocal about the issues that affect them.

The process of sexual arousal is similar in women to that in men. In women, the engorgement of the sexual organs (the clitoris and the inner and outer labia round the vagina), and lubrication by internal secretions, all happen via nervous system activity. This process is an aid not just to sexual intercourse, but also to sexual pleasure. Given that the nervous system controlling urination, bowel activity and leg mobility may be damaged, control of the process of engorgement – parallel to the process of erection in men – may well be affected. Sensations in the genital area may be also affected.

Artificial lubrication, with a lubricant such as K-Y Jelly, can deal with problems of vaginal dryness. However, whilst such lubrication may allow sexual intercourse more easily, it may well not deal with the complex range of other issues that surround sexual arousal and fulfilment in women, and these should be dealt with in the future in the same increasingly sensitive and sympathetic way as those of men.

I really don't feel like having sex any more. Is this the result of the MS? I am worried that my relationship with my husband is now deteriorating badly as a result. What can I do?

It is often difficult to disentangle the various changes that may occur as a result of MS from other factors. Sometimes symptoms like depression or fatigue which are indirect (or secondary) symptoms of MS, may play as large a part in the way that you feel sexually as primary neurological damage. If such symptoms are treated successfully then your sexual drive (often called your *libido*) may increase.

If the main cause of your decreasing sexual drive lies in primary neurological damage, then this is harder to deal with directly. You and your husband could perhaps consider other means of having a sensual set of experiences, without you feeling the immediate pressure for sexual intercourse – other parts of your body may be more erotically sensitive. With gentle mutual touch and exploration you may find, as many other couples have done both with and without MS, that you can introduce a new sensual and loving element into your relationship. Make time to enjoy the experiences with each other without feeling hurried or under pressure. Such an approach may bring about a new, different but satisfying relationship with your partner. Most relationships involve planning – it is just that with MS a little more planning is required.

I've heard a lot about Viagra for men's impotence recently. Could that help me sexually?

There has been an enormous amount of publicity about Viagra in recent months, and the ways in which it may transform people's – especially men's – sexual lives. Fortunately for many men with erection problems, caused by nervous system damage in MS, it may indeed offer some assistance.

Essentially Viagra acts on the blood supply problems in MS, by helping the penis to fill with blood. Even where nervous system damage is substantial and where erections are very difficult to obtain and sustain, Viagra may be able to assist such problems.

At present the drug is taken orally (by mouth) and, because of the relatively slow digestive process, it may be an hour or two before the drug produces its effects – certainly an issue in planning sexual activity. It affects not just the penile area, but has potential effects all over the body. There may, therefore, be some side effects elsewhere, so your cardiovascular health will be assessed before Viagra is prescribed. As with most drugs, not everyone will benefit, although Viagra has been found to produce firmer, more frequent and longer lasting erections in the majority of men who have taken it.

Men who are taking medications for heart conditions, such as nitrates, which help to lower blood pressure, run the risk of a dangerous further drop in blood pressure in taking Viagra. Older men, perhaps with an underlying undiagnosed cardiac problem, who may not have undertaken any exercise for several years, could find themselves in difficulty with vigorous sexual activity, so it is important that you discuss things fully with your doctor. However, as many men with MS are in younger age groups than those in which major side effects with Viagra have occurred, there should be fewer problems amongst those men.

Note that because of the cost of the drug, and the assumed large demand for it, the Department of Health has been extremely circumspect about those for whom it can be prescribed via the NHS. However, MS is now one of the designated medical conditions – but there may still be local variations in supply, in addition to clinical reasons for its non-prescription.

Could women with MS benefit from Viagra as well?

As we noted earlier, there are some very similar processes occurring in women to those in men, so in theory Viagra could help to enhance sexual pleasure, but there have been few systematic studies of women's sexual response while on the drug, and none completed as yet in relation to women with MS. Women may feel that this again shows very particular gender bias in the testing of such drugs! Such studies are now being undertaken.

I have a problem with incontinence. This is proving to be difficult for me to manage in any case, but particularly so when I want to have sex with my husband. Is there anything I can do?

You should already have had a careful and recent assessment of the problems you have with incontinence, and have received the best available advice on the most comfortable ways of managing them. If you have not, you should seek such an assessment through your doctor. Try and ensure that you have no urinary infections, which can make your bladder problems worse if left untreated. You should be particularly careful about this issue and constantly on the lookout for any infection. Discuss your concerns with your husband because, by doing so, you may feel less anxious and, if he thinks that you are doing all you can to minimize the problems, then he may be much more positive than you fear.

There are other things you can do to help reduce the risk of 'accidents' during intercourse:

- Reduce your intake of fluids for an hour or two beforehand.

- If you are self-catheterizing, do so shortly before you begin.

- If you are taking drugs to reduce urgency because of a bladder storage problem, take these about 30 minutes beforehand to ensure as far as possible that no spontaneous bladder contractions occur.

- You may need to ensure more vaginal lubrication, with something such as K-Y Jelly.

- Check out gently and sensitively positions in which you both feel comfortable, and in which you feel you are less likely to have problems with leakage.

- If you have an in-dwelling catheter, then several positions may be better than others (remember also to empty the collecting bag, and tape the catheter to your body to prevent it moving): a rear entry position may be easiest to manage, lying on your side with your partner behind you; or, while he kneels, lie on your back with your legs over his shoulders.

When we had sex recently, I found it a painful experience. What can I do?

Usually the problem here is insufficient vaginal lubrication. Low levels of sexual arousal can reduce lubrication, but it can also be due to damage to nerve pathways in the mid- and upper spinal cord area, which leads to inadequate stimulation of the lower nerve pathways to the genital area; certain drugs taken for other purposes – such as urinary problems – also dry up vaginal secretions. Sometimes lubrication can be assisted by direct stimulation of the genital area; or try to set up an environment which is as relaxing and conducive to sexual thoughts and experiences. As far as additional lubrication is concerned, K-Y Jelly or a similar water-soluble substance can be very helpful. Substances like Vaseline are not recommended because they do not dissolve in water, and they are likely to leave residues which could give rise to infections. They can also create holes and tears in condoms.

The spasticity in my legs proved to be a big problem when I tried to have sexual intercourse recently. Is there any advice you can offer me about this?

The effect of unexpected spasms in your legs, or elsewhere, during sexual activity, can be very disconcerting. The important thing is to check with your doctor that the general control of your spasticity is as good as it can be. The normal approach to spasticity is to try and keep your muscles as well toned as possible through regular exercises (see Chapter 10), and to use appropriate drugs such as baclofen as necessary to give additional control.

There are also certain positions for sexual activity which appear to make the muscular spasms less likely, although it is important that you explore other possibilities than those mentioned below, for you may find a position that suits you both very well, which is not described here. For a man who may have difficulty with spasms or rigidity in his legs, then sitting in an appropriate chair (without arms) would allow his partner to sit on his penis either facing him or with her back to him. For a woman, lying on her side may help, perhaps with a towel or other

material between your legs for more comfort. Your partner can
then approach you from behind. Another possibility is to lie on
your back towards the edge of your bed with the lower part of
your legs hanging loosely off the bed.

**Fatigue is my major problem when it comes to sex. I just
don't feel I have the energy.**

Many people with MS find that fatigue is a problem with a great
many of their activities, owing to its often unpredictable nature.
As with other symptoms associated with MS, it is important to
discuss this with your doctor who will assess the best means of
managing it, which is not easy. Although there are one or two
drugs which may help (for example amantadine or pemoline)
and which – if prescribed for you – might be taken a few minutes
before sexual activity, currently the best help is through various
appropriate lifestyle changes. Fatigue is discussed in further
detail in Chapter 9.

One obvious way forward is to consider at what times you feel
least fatigued. Although this may not necessarily be the time
when you feel that you should be having sex – such as in the
morning, or during the day, rather than at a more conventional
time – you may be less tired and enjoy it more. Rather than thinking of sexual intercourse as the major element, you could agree
with your partner to engage in some other less energetic sexual
activities – such as gentle stroking or foreplay – that you could
participate in more frequently. As with so many other aspects of
living with MS, it is a question of finding ways to adapt to the situation through experimentation.

**I feel I am unusual as someone with MS who is gay. Almost
all the advice I read about sexuality and MS implies that
people are heterosexual and are in opposite sex partner-
ships. Is there any recognition of the problems that
people like me face?**

You are quite right that, until recently, it has not been recognized
at all that some people with MS are gay. Even in the increasing

material that is being written about sexuality and disabled people, the particular problems of being gay are often not covered. According to national surveys, perhaps 1 in 10 people with MS are gay, so there may be many people with MS who feel as you do.

The MS Society has recently established a lesbian and gay group. Details may be obtained from the national MS Society. For disabled and non-disabled lesbian and bisexual women, there is an organization called GEMMA, and it would also be worth contacting SPOD (the Association to Aid the Sexual and Personal Relationships of People with a Disability) for further information and advice (see Appendix 1 for addresses).

I have MS, and am young and single, and most of the information available on sexuality seems to be for people who are in long-term relationships with another person. Can you give me any advice?

Yes, it is often assumed that the majority of the population both with and without MS is already in a stable, usually married, long-term relationship. In fact, there are many people like yourself, including those who have divorced or whose relationships have broken down, an increasing number of single parents, and those whose partner has died. We live in a society where people are in increasingly many different forms of relationship to others. Gradually the information available for people with MS is reflecting this situation.

Do realize that you are not alone with whatever problems you may have, even though it sometimes seems as though most of what is written for people with MS assumes you are already in a relationship with someone else. Much of the advice in this section in the questions on sexual problems and sexual responsiveness is equally applicable to single people.

14
Pregnancy and childbirth

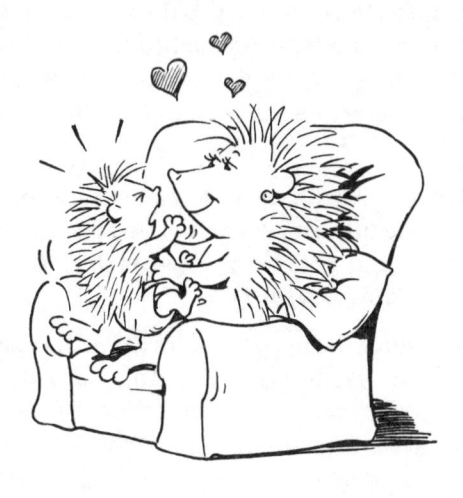

Issues concerning pregnancy and childbirth often worry people with MS and their partners, as many such people will have recently embarked on relationships in which they will be considering the possibility of having children. Bringing up children is also another area which concerns both people with MS and those close to them. We discuss in this chapter questions often raised in relation to these issues.

I have just been diagnosed with MS. What will the effect on my MS be if I had a baby?

Many women may be worried about possible short-term consequences of the MS during the pregnancy and immediately after the birth, and also about possible long-term consequences for the MS itself in having a child. We can be reassuring about the consequences of MS in pregnancy itself; if anything, the evidence is that rates of relapse are lower at this time, and many women feel freer of symptoms than they have for some time. There is also no evidence that the long-term course of MS is any different for those women who have been pregnant than those who haven't. There is, however, research showing that in the six months after the birth more women than we would otherwise expect do have a relapse – perhaps between a quarter and a third of all women. Unfortunately there is no way to predict whether you will yourself be one of those women.

Although I have discussed the situation with my GP and neurologist, I am concerned about what my obstetrician might say about being pregnant with MS?

There are still some doctors – neurologists and obstetricians amongst them – who may still advise someone with MS not to become pregnant, or to have a termination. You may find that some members of your family or others share that view, often based on outdated information as to how pregnancy and child-birth affects MS. The significant point is that you feel you can discuss both your plans and any worries you have with doctors, and other professional staff looking after you. Pregnancy and childbirth is a time when it is important to have continuing sup-port from, as well as trust in, those helping you. You can receive good support and advice, and possibly information about sympa-thetic obstetricians, from the local branch of the MS Society or other MS support group.

What sort of issues would you advise someone with MS to consider before becoming pregnant?

Having a child is a very individual decision, and although in the past there was often very clear and very negative advice given about pregnancy to someone with MS by medical and other pro-fessional staff, in general this view has changed. The issue is not so much about educating women with MS towards not having a child but providing information about all aspects of pregnancy and child care, so that an informed choice can be made. The issues concerned in becoming pregnant are those for the most part which would concern all women and their partners – about coping with the pregnancy and childbirth itself; future issues of parenting; the effect on relationships, and the additional financial costs that would be incurred and so on. An added problem is, of course, the relatively unpredictable nature of MS. A useful way to proceed is to discuss with your partner and/or family and close friends, a series of 'What if?' questions, considering, for example, some of the problems that might occur financially or in relation to child care. Through these means you can rehearse some of the ways of managing potential difficulties, in the hope, and in many cases the expectation, that such problems will not occur.

Is it likely that a woman with MS will have any additional risks or problems in pregnancy or childbirth itself?

The answer in general is no. We have already indicated that relapses tend to be lower in number during pregnancy, and over-all most women find their pregnancy is relatively uneventful from an MS point of view. In childbirth itself, some women with MS who have muscular weakness in their legs or lower bodies, or who may have spasms, might need some assistance with childbirth – perhaps an epidural anaesthesia, for example, or the use of forceps or even a caesarean. However, there is little evidence that MS causes major additional changes in the way that babies are delivered compared to those of women without MS.

The overall advice for women with MS in relation to preparing for the birth is also the same for all women: prenatal classes, run by your local midwives, and often also by the National Childbirth Trust, would be useful both for you and your partner to attend, if you have one, so that you can be taken through the stages of labour and how best to manage them. It may help to discuss techniques of pain relief with your midwife and the obstetrician.

Another point you may need to know concerns steroids. If you have been taking steroids over the past few months, such as Prednisone (generic name prednisolone) – and this is one of the drugs that pregnant women have taken safely – then it is possible during the delivery that you will need an extra dose of this drug. This is because, during labour, the adrenal gland may be 'overloaded' if you have taken steroid drugs over the preceding months, and an additional dose, a 'boost', is needed. Raise this issue with your midwife and the obstetrician before the delivery itself, so that they are aware of the situation.

I am currently taking several drugs to combat the effects of the MS. Do I need to stop taking these, if I decide to become pregnant?

As an important general rule you should not take any drug, even an over-the-counter drug, during pregnancy, or indeed when you are considering becoming pregnant, without discussing this first with your doctor, and receiving his or her advice on the possible consequences for your pregnancy. For many drugs used to treat the everyday symptoms of MS, there is substantial information available about the consequences of their use during pregnancy, and many of them are safe to use – but you do need to check each one with your doctor. Those drugs which are now being used to treat the disease itself, rather than any one specific symptom, such as the interferon-based drugs (such as Avonex, Betaferon and Rebif) and Copaxone, are powerful immunosuppressants, and it is still not entirely clear what effects they will have on an unborn baby. Until the position is clear, or unless otherwise advised to do so by your doctor, it would be wise to suspend taking such drugs once you have started trying for a baby, for it will be some time before you know you are pregnant, and in the meantime the fertilized egg could be developing. It is a question of balancing your own concerns about the effects of MS on you, and the health of your unborn baby. The decision may not be easy one to make, but most mothers treat the health of their unborn baby as their main concern at this time. If you decide not to breastfeed your baby, you can start taking these drugs again shortly after the delivery of the baby. If you decide to breastfeed, then you do need to seek your doctor's advice – for drugs may be passed to the baby in breast milk.

If a relapse is possible after giving birth, should I have a baby?

It is still only a minority of women with MS who may have a relapse in the six months after the birth. In addition, given the advent of the newer interferon-based drugs or copolymer (Copaxone) it is possible, after discussions with your neurologist, that you can take one of those drugs – which are known to reduce the chances of a relapse – immediately after the birth (but see the answer below to the question on breastfeeding). In any case, as we have said, the longer term outlook for you is no different than that for women not having a baby; the increased likelihood of a relapse is only in those first few months after the birth. Furthermore, having a baby involves many decisions, irrespective of the presence of MS, and such consequences are likely to weigh as heavily, perhaps even more so, than the effects of MS immediately after the birth.

What about breastfeeding? Is that going to have any effect on my MS?

Breastfeeding is generally recognized as giving the baby the best possible food in the first few months. However, doctors, especially neurologists, used to advise women with MS against breastfeeding. This was mainly because it was thought that breastfeeding produced an additional strain on such women, and might even precipitate a relapse. However, there is little evidence that breastfeeding in itself has any harmful effects like this. If you feel you are able to breastfeed, with helpful advice or assistance from your midwife, health visitor or doctor, then you should do so.

Of course breastfeeding is only a part of an often exhausting experience that all women have in caring for a newborn baby. If you can, arrange for someone else to help you in the first few weeks after the birth, and whilst it is important – if you wish to continue breastfeeding – to undertake all the feeding yourself in the first two or three weeks, someone else could help with the particularly exhausting night-time feeds with previously expressed breast milk, or with a relevant formula feed.

Just to reiterate, it is important to be very careful about drugs you are taking during breastfeeding, for they may be passed to the baby through breast milk. With the newer interferon-based drugs and copolymer (Copaxone), you must seek your doctor's advice if you are breastfeeding. In the present uncertain state of knowledge about their effects on breastfed babies, you may have to consider not breastfeeding your baby, if you take these drugs.

15
You and your family

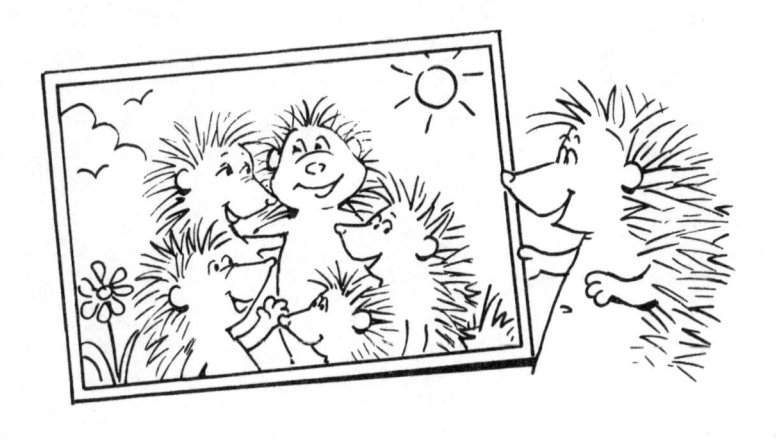

Relationships with partners and family members

Managing relationships with partners is difficult even without the presence of MS. How much MS itself affects such relationships is always hard to judge precisely, because of the many different kinds of relationships that exist between two people. Of course MS does bring complications of its own, sometimes major ones that have to be dealt with, but it often highlights the positive and the negative aspects of relationships which were already there.

With my MS everything seems to be so uncertain from day to day, even from minute to minute. My husband doesn't really understand. Is there anything we can do to help each other?

As you imply, the uncertainties linked with MS are difficult to manage, for both of you. On the one hand, the 'hidden' symptoms of MS, such as fatigue and continence problems, can appear at any time, thus placing you in a situation where you may not be able to plan even more than a few minutes ahead in relation to your daily activities. On the other hand, your life with MS requires planning to ensure that when you do things, both inside and outside the home, you can make the best possible arrangements to ensure that you can do them well. All this will often be very frustrating.

Although the longer term future with MS is uncertain, the key daily problem for many people like yourself is managing their fatigue. As we have noted in Chapter 9, working out your own daily 'fatigue cycle' as best you can, and pacing your activities involving your husband in relation to that, can help a lot. You may have been prescribed one of the relevant drugs (such as amantadine) to help. However, being realistic, current drug therapies for MS fatigue are for the most part unlikely to produce the major changes which many people with MS hope for, so the main strategy will be to get to know your own daily rhythms and events.

The key thing as far as your husband is concerned is to try and get him to appreciate that the variability in your symptoms is not your fault or under your direct control. This is sometimes difficult, for even those people who know you well may feel sometimes that, when you say you are too tired to do something you have planned, you are 'putting it on'. It might help if your husband were to read a bit more about MS (perhaps this book), or to discuss this issue with your GP, neurologist or another health professional who knows the effects of MS well. He should then be able to see that the uncertainties and changes in your symptoms are due to the MS, and that you are equally as frustrated as he is about them.

We know that, in some families, the problems associated with MS become such a major focus that relationships can break down. It is important to work out ways of sharing or developing other mutual interests, involving less physical activity perhaps, before this happens. Tell your husband about services that are available for 'carers' (see the section below on *Being a carer*) so that he knows he is not alone in his feelings and problems.

I suppose you could say I've always been a 'houseproud' person, and wanted to make a good home for my husband and myself. I really feel our relationship is now in difficulties because with my MS I can't keep the house going as I should. What should I do?

Relationships are built on all kinds of different things. However, despite modern attitudes, looking after the home well is still something which many women, and often their partners feel is important. It may be difficult to deal with a situation where it becomes hard for you to do this, but it would be very unusual for a relationship to be built only on looking after the home well – there will be other things that you like and share in common. We talk about prioritizing jobs like housework in Chapter 9. Maybe you could afford someone to come in for an hour or two a week, and undertake tasks which are important but difficult for you to do, or perhaps have a home help for a few hours. Some women find having someone doing household tasks for them quite difficult – even if they can afford it – because they think it undermines their role further but, if you can think of that help as releasing you to do other things with your husband which you would be too tired to do without that help, then this might make you feel better about the situation.

Both my partner and myself have always looked after ourselves, and people say what an attractive couple we make, but I really am worried that the MS will ruin our relationship.

MS often affects people when they are young. They may worry that things like looks and physical achievements, which younger people value more, will be totally lost. Apart from some unusual situations when the MS proceeds very rapidly, it is likely to be some time before there are very visible long-term bodily effects. In the longer term, of course, everyone with or without MS has to adjust to the effects of ageing!

Relationships with children

My 6-year-old girl says she is worried that she might get MS, now that she has seen her mummy with the condition.

Although children may worry about this, their anxiety may not emerge explicitly in family discussions. In Chapter 3, we talk about the inherited component in MS. The risk is very small so you should be very reassuring. You should also reassure your daughter on another point, that MS is not 'catching' or

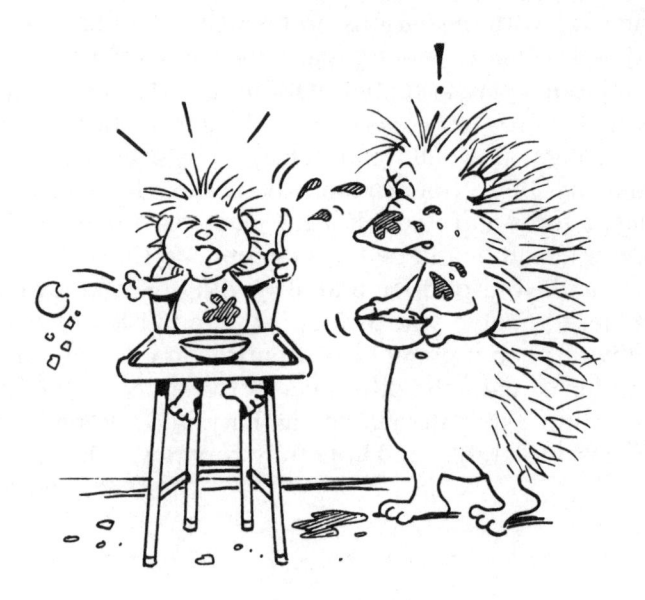

contagious. Sometimes children feel anything that is, in their experience, out of the ordinary, may be 'catching', largely because so many adult discussions with children about health, talk about problems of 'catching' illnesses from other people – both from adults and children.

At first I was concerned about the possibility of passing on my MS to my children. Now my main concern is being able to bring them up as I should. Will I be able to do this properly?

Of course it depends what you mean by 'properly'! Most future parents are very committed to wanting the best for their child, and have clear views about what they want to avoid as well as how they want to be parents. It is quite right that they have those ambitions, but most parents find, in practice, that their world with children is more complicated, less predictable and less easy to manage than planned: relationships between partners break down; jobs change or are lost and money can be tight, so compromises have to be made. In addition, children, as most parents find, have minds and wishes of their own!

Having MS, with the various problems it might bring in parenting, is just one factor among many that may affect the bringing up of children. Do not feel that without the MS parenting of children would somehow be easier, or indeed turn out well, although clearly having young children is a major physical burden in terms of managing their hour-to-hour activities, feeding, wayward sleeping patterns and so on. For the early years of a child's life, it is important, as it would be for all people, to think through daily activities with your partner, and also with other family members if possible, to enable you to feel that the burden of daily child care activities is not going to rest entirely on you. Such support in the end may make the difference between feeling child care is an almost impossibly demanding activity, and feeling that it is at the very least tolerable, and hopefully very rewarding.

I have two young children who are not yet of school age. How much should I tell them about my MS?

Many parents worry about when and how to tell their children that they have MS. Such a view is often based on a misunderstanding of what a child, even a very young one, is likely to have observed, or even to have understood. Children are very acute observers, and almost certainly will have picked up on any anxieties – about MS as well as other things – some time before you think they have. They may not know what exactly 'MS' is, but will probably already be aware that mummy or daddy may find difficulty in doing some things, or that there are heated (or hushed) discussions about other things to do with everyday life. In such a situation, when the opportunity arises, perhaps when you are trying to do a particularly difficult task, then a matter-of-fact, non-technical and brief explanation as to how the difficulty has arisen will be helpful, however young the children are. Over time, these explanations can be elaborated. The key thing is to treat the MS, as almost certainly you do yourself, as an everyday issue, rather than one with mountainous implications for the future, which may upset your children.

Children may well ask questions themselves such as 'Why did you nearly fall over then?' or 'Why are you wobbly?' or 'Why are you walking with a stick?' If this happens, you could answer, depending on their age, by talking about your illness which means that your legs don't always move as well as they should, because messages to your leg muscles from your brain don't always get through. This makes you wobbly and you have to use a stick (or wheelchair) to help you. You can say more about MS itself, or indeed about other symptoms, on other occasions, or when they ask for more detail.

Although parents may try understandably to protect their children from what the parents see as the disturbing aspects of MS, young children may think that there is a major family secret not being discussed with them, and which is very threatening – precisely because it is not talked through. Fears might include the early death of the parent with MS, or indeed their own deaths. You should be reassuring about both these aspects.

To be generally reassuring, talk about the MS with your children as though it is a part – although only a part – of their lives, as it is of yours. Explain things as each situation arises, especially when children themselves are curious or ask questions. If children feel you are being honest in responding to their questions or concerns, both you and they are less likely to have problems later.

My 12-year-old son seems to feel that he is responsible for my MS, and keeps on worrying about us looking after him: he thinks he is a burden on us. How can I reassure him?

Many children, particularly those who are under pressure or who feel very sensitive about MS in their family or its consequences, may feel responsible for the MS by having been 'naughty' in the past. They often don't explicitly say this to their parents – at least in your case you are aware of your son's feelings. Be reassuring about this point, and ensure that your son is aware that, whatever he may or may not have done, this had no bearing on your MS. Of course some mothers may have (mistakenly) blamed their MS itself, or some of its symptoms, on a pregnancy and the associated childbirth – it is possible that this feeling has been picked up by a child!

The fact that your son feels he is a burden on you needs some mutual discussion, to ascertain why he feels this way, and how best to manage these feelings. Often – to parents' surprise – children do feel as responsible for their parents, as their parents feel responsible for them, particularly if there appears to be some problem – such as long-term illness – which is causing difficulties in their family. Allow your son to express his concern for you, and show your appreciation of that concern, but also reassure him that he is not a burden on you in the way he thinks, and is loved for being himself. Try to agree some small ways in which he can help by doing some specific jobs in the house, for example. This can help him feel that he is contributing to the family.

My daughter is in her final A level year in her sixth form college, and I assumed that she would go to University – which we should like her to do. However, although she applied, and has already obtained a place at a University several hours' journey from our home, she now tells me that she doesn't want to go, and at the same time says how worried she is about me.

There could be several reasons for this. Although many young people like your daughter do go to University, others have different plans – at least immediately after they have left school – and will take up a job without going to University, or perhaps postpone their entry until a little later in life. As Universities and Colleges are now much more geared to admitting and supporting what they describe as 'mature' students, going to University later in life should not prove a major problem from that point of view.

However, as your daughter has linked her wish that she now doesn't want to go to University with her concern for you, it does seem that there may be issues here to do with your MS. It is important to tell her that you want her to go to University, without putting undue pressure on her. You need to reassure her that you do not think it is her role, or duty to look after you; at the same time indicate how you propose to deal with any further disability that may develop – this will reassure her that you have been thinking about such issues yourself. She may be worried also about your – and her – financial position at University. Be as reassuring as you can, and perhaps seek advice yourself about likely financial issues, to be better informed yourself, before speaking to her. The main aim here is to give as much acknowledgement as possible to her views, ambitions and concerns, and to indicate that her priorities are as important as those of others in the family.

I am very concerned at my situation. My husband left me three years ago and, as my MS has got worse, I have become very dependent on my 14-year-old daughter to

**help me with all kinds of things, such as washing me and
helping me to the toilet.**

The issue of 'young carers' is one which has come to public
attention more and more over the past few years. It is a complex
issue. People who do not know your situation might think that
your daughter is 'losing her childhood or early adolescence' and
wish to have her removed from the tasks that you describe, and
her general caring role, immediately. Such an immediate reaction
might produce an even more difficult situation. It is important to
try and achieve a balanced view of how to proceed.

The key issue is how children can help but still ensure their
own futures through doing well in formal education, and through
play and leisure in their own time. Try and get help with your
personal care more from other adults, either in your household or
professionally. Unfortunately, support available for young carers
is as variable as for other forms of service provision for people
with MS, so you will need to press for it, or find a friendly
professional person you know or a robust friend to act as an
'advocate' for you and your daughter. The MS Society is aware of
these issues, and the Carers' National Association has a special
interest in the support of young carers, and should be able to
offer advice and support (see Appendices 1 and 2).

**My son, who is now 15, doesn't do a thing in the house
or help me. He wants to go out with his friends all the
time, many of whom we don't approve. My wife and I have
tried hard to bring him up well, but we are now in despair
about him.**

We can hear many parents saying the same thing as you, even
without MS in the family! Bringing up children, and particularly
teenagers, is a problem for any family. It is difficult to know how
much your son has reacted to your MS, or whether there are
other factors involved. However, the early and mid-teen years
are when young people of both sexes are beginning to assert
their independence from their family – often generating difficult
and fraught family relationships. This is a necessary part of

'growing up', which family members, and particularly parents, may have difficulty acknowledging. Exactly what effects the addition of MS have in any individual family setting is difficult to judge.

It may be that he is just 'being a teenager' or he may feel too much pressure to stay at home and help, which will curb his freedom even more. Although you are undoubtedly under considerable pressure yourself, the only way this is likely to be resolved is through patience and tolerance. You could seek some informal advice and support from other parents in a similar situation, for example in your local MS Society branch, or consult your doctor about a possible referral for family therapy where all the members of the family could talk through the situation and consider ways forward.

As a man with MS I am really concerned about my role in disciplining my children. I am not very mobile at the moment, but I want them to know that I am still 'in charge'.

The issue of disciplining children is a tricky and difficult one for parents with MS, and particularly for fathers. There are different styles of discipline, some more forceful and direct than others. The more effective your expertise in negotiation and communication the less likely it will be that you have to resort to direct discipline of a more verbal or even a physical kind.

Because some fathers cannot join in with physical games and activities, particularly with sons, they try and assert their authority in other ways. However, remember that children are very adaptable. You might have a good knowledge of sport, or you could participate in other things in which they are interested. Nevertheless, all children need to see where the boundaries lie, but if the boundaries are always drawn in a fiercely robust and negative rather than positive way, then you may be storing up some problems for the future. Challenging behaviour may underlie his fears about you and your MS, and this may require quite a different response.

Don't forget that parenting, including disciplining children, should be undertaken with the help of others, including partners and family members. Don't feel that you have to do it all on your own.

As a woman with MS I really do feel I am exhausted when my children come home from school. They want my attention, and want to show me things and involve me in all the things they do – but often I just haven't the energy.

Fatigue associated with MS is often a problem, and as we have noted in Chapter 9, a combination of a careful assessment of your own daily patterns of fatigue, and possibly some medication from your doctor, will help you plan the day a bit better, so that you can include the children more in your activities.

Other mothers with MS usually deal with these problems by pacing activities during the earlier part of the day. You can then rest before the children come home from school. If you are working outside the home, then again it is important, if you can, to schedule a time where you can relax and rest before giving your attention to your children. Try and discuss the problem with your children, so that they are aware that you want to find a way in which you can have regular and dedicated time together. You could perhaps put together a combination of 'time slots' with slightly less demanding activities. This may provide other benefits as well, in the form of closer ties with your children, and their understanding of you and your difficulties.

Once or twice my daughter – who is now 11 years old – has been a little late for school because I haven't been able to get everything ready for her in the morning, and from time to time she has had to help me. Should I let the school know about my MS?

In most circumstances it is important that you do so. You do not say, and maybe you do not know, what reasons your daughter has given to the school when she has been late. As schools are becoming more concerned about pupils' punctuality, it is a good idea to let at least her class teacher know about your situation.

The school may arrange a discussion with her teacher, so that any questions or concerns that the teacher may have about MS, as well as any consequences for your daughter, could be discussed. You can address the issue of occasional lateness, and you will be also reassured that the teacher understands MS and its effects more accurately. If you can establish a good and collaborative relationship with your daughter's main class or form teacher, it is likely that you will all benefit. Your daughter will probably not want to be seen by her peers or her teachers as someone who is 'very different' from others in her class, and so you should be sensitive to her worries about how these discussions are handled at the school.

Being a carer

I am really annoyed with the word 'carer' when it's applied to me. I suppose I am doing the caring, but he's my husband and I'm not just a carer.

Some people do have negative feelings about the word 'carer' – they feel like a 'one-dimensional' person, that it implies they have no life or interests of their own. On the other hand, others feel that being called a 'carer' is much more positive, for it recognizes the many things that you do for the person with MS, which can be just taken for granted. Of course, increasingly there are services and support targeted at 'carers'. You should take advantage of those services, even if it means, for these purposes, that you are considered a carer.

It is very important that everybody, from friends to professionals, recognizes that your relationship with your husband is more complex than caring alone, and that you have your own interests, ideas and concerns. Make sure that you have time to yourself so that you can 'recharge your batteries' outside the daily and often onerous demands of being a carer.

I really feel my life is a constant battle for services and support for my wife. Nothing seems easy or simple to obtain.

This is a very common complaint by family members of people with MS. Part of the problem is often that there seems to be no central source of information which can be used to access those services that you need, now and possibly later. You will need to experiment to find out what is the best source in your area.

Your local MS Society can put you in touch with others in a similar situation, and the National MS Society arranges regional meetings for carers. At a more general level, the Carers National Association may be able to tell you whether there are services in your area, and produce many leaflets to help you get the best out of services on offer. Otherwise, your local Social Services Department or local library should know of it (see Appendices 1 and 2.

The Community Care Act requires that Social Services Departments make available information about services in their area. If your wife has been assessed by your local Social Services Department, then she should have been allocated a care manager who will also be helpful as a source of information and support. Some other authorities are establishing key workers, who should be able to offer a similar level of support. Respite care is dealt with in Chapter 12.

16
Other relationships

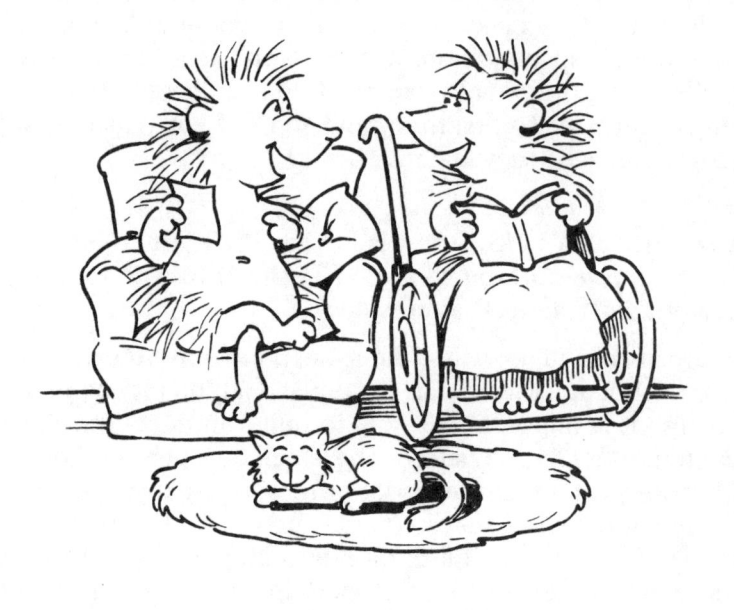

Relationships with friends

**My friends often tell me how well I look – even when
I'm feeling bad – and it's even worse when I am having a
really bad day and using my wheelchair. I sometimes hear
whispers like 'Why is he in a wheelchair? He looks OK'.
What can I do?**

People in general often have particular views about what others
'should' look like when they have a serious or long-term illness.

Most of these views are based on common ideas about how people appear when they have infectious diseases (like influenza, pneumonia or measles), or heart conditions, or when they are very old. Those with conditions like MS, and a number of other neurological conditions, often do not look 'ill' in this way at all. There may be opportunities sometimes to explain to others how you really do feel and let them know that 'looks aren't everything'. You could explain how difficult is to walk as your muscles are difficult to control, or how your eyesight is a problem. You may need to explain more about MS, and that it is also a long-term condition, and so won't just 'go away' as an infectious disease usually does. Of course, people may be just trying to lift your spirits, to try and support you – as they would do for others who they feel may be ill.

Since I have had MS, I feel it is very difficult to make friends. I'm beginning to feel that the future is looking bleak socially as well as physically.

You are still, in many ways, the same person as you were before the MS. Although the MS has introduced a difficult component in your life, it is important for you to build on those things which were important to you before. There will be a period of time, and perhaps especially in the period after being diagnosed, when it may be difficult to re-orientate yourself to the new circumstances. It may be helpful to talk through positive ways forward with someone close to you, or perhaps a counsellor, or others with MS who may be going through the same process as yourself. If you present yourself as a person with a rich range of ideas, attitudes and opinions that you have developed through your life, then others will like you. Not everyone of course, but then few of us make friends with everyone.

Should I tell other people I meet about my diagnosis? My symptoms are not yet very obvious to people who don't know me, but I always feel that I have to tell others at some time.

When you tell people about your MS depends very much on who they are and the situation involved. There really is no single strategy. When and how you tell some people – such as employers – could have significant effects on your job and career. We discuss this issue in Chapter 12.

If the MS has a significant impact on your life, then it will be very difficult not to tell other people at some point. However, you may need to be prepared for several types of reactions. Remember that telling people will always occur in a dialogue with them, and they will not only listen to the words you say, but also how you say them, as well as your general demeanour. If you make a special point of telling people when you first meet them, and appear very awkward or very earnest about your MS, then you are likely to get different responses than if you appear to be treating MS as just a part of your life. Try telling other people when the conversation turns to symptoms or illnesses, or what they are able or not able to do.

Be prepared to answer questions about what MS is and how it affects you. People's initial reactions may, of course, mask their own concern about how to respond as much as anything else.

I had a very busy social life before I was diagnosed with MS – indeed problems in keeping up with my previously hectic social life was one reason I knew something was wrong. Now I am trying to keep everything going, and I'm finding it very difficult. Am I going to lose my friends?

Given the pressures of various combinations of social, family and work commitments, many people find that there is not only not enough time in the day to do everything, but fatigue – or other symptoms – set in and further limit what they can really do. Although it may not seem like it, if you think seriously about the balance of the things you do, you will probably find that you can prioritize your various activities.

You might also need to plan some periods of time when you can relax and rest, which may initially be frustrating to you, but necessary to maintain your other commitments. Such commitments, and the people associated with them, then can be made

more special, and they will appreciate the fact that you have
made them a priority.

Relationships with the medical profession

In the course of MS and its treatment, people with MS – and their
relatives – often have questions and concerns about their relationship to their medical and health practitioners. In this section,
we address some these worries.

**Now I know that I have MS, who is really responsible for
looking after me?**

Your GP is medically responsible for your general, routine day-
to-day health care. Most GPs will refer you on clinical grounds to
support services for people with MS, often in the practice itself,
such as nursing, counselling and, possibly, physiotherapy. Some
larger general practices are also setting up multidisciplinary
support clinics for patients with long-term conditions which,
although not specifically targeted to MS, could be of value to
people with the disease.

However, once you have been referred to, and then been
diagnosed by, a consultant (usually a neurologist), you are now
automatically his or her patient as well. Thus, in principle,
someone with MS could have an embarrassment of services, in
both general practice and in a hospital setting! However, this not
usually the case. One of the major problems at present is that
services are patchily distributed and relatively ill-coordinated,
and people with MS are having to take what is available to them.
In the light of this unsatisfactory situation, the MS Society and
leading neurologists have recently put together a minimum
standard of service provision for people with MS which they hope
will lead to more consistent provision (see Appendix 2).

Technically the GP and the specialist should be in touch with one another, informing each other of developments in relation to your health. This does not always happen efficiently. The best advice is to use whichever local services are most convenient and helpful for whatever problems you happen to have, and to press your GP and/or the consultant as necessary for other services that you feel have not been offered. The advent of MS clinics with other professional staff, such as nurses, as primary advisers may provide more support in due course.

I don't feel I am getting along very well with my GP, I don't think she understands me or my MS. Can I change to another GP?

In theory you can change your GP at any time simply by registering with another GP. Obviously if you cannot form an effective working relationship with your GP, then this is a good last resort, but building a rapport with any doctor may take a great deal of time and effort by both parties. MS itself is not an easy condition to manage, in that it throws up many symptoms over its course that can need considerable medical attention or advice. Thus, for a hard-pressed GP, you may be considered to be rather a demanding patient. Whilst this should not put you off from consulting your GP for symptoms that worry you, it may be sensible to consider other sources of medical advice and support where possible. These could include nurses in the GP's practice; an MS clinic if one is available at your local hospital; or possibly your neurologist, although an appointment may take a considerable time to arrange.

If you still wish to change your GP, then in practice this depends on whether you can find another GP who is willing to take you. In most areas of the UK, this is unlikely to be a problem, although it may involve some time on the telephone, and you do need to bear in mind that a potential GP will have to take into account that you may be a heavy user of his or her time and the practice services. However, if there is any difficulty in changing your GP, you should consult your local Health Authority which oversees the operation of health services in each area.

Can I ask for a second opinion without upsetting my doctor?

Second opinions are an important part of all clinical practice, and doctors will review cases with their colleagues as a matter of course. If you wish to seek a second opinion, then you can do so through your GP, who should provide a referral and possibly make the appointment on your behalf. It is not likely that simply asking for a second opinion will upset any doctor.

What tips would you give me for getting the most out of my visit to my doctor?

- Ask for an explanation of any words that you don't understand – including illnesses, medicines, symptoms or treatments.

- Ask what results you can expect from any drugs, therapies or medications given to you. Should you expect only a little or a more significant change in your condition? When should these changes occur?

- Ask about any other options that you might have and their advantages or disadvantages.

- Ask about side effects that you might have from any drugs or therapies prescribed for you.

- Ask about any follow-up procedures. When and on what basis will you be seen next time?

- Before a visit to your doctor, write anything down that you need to ask, noting important points that you don't want to forget to discuss.

- Note down important points arising from your discussions with your doctor as soon as possible. Increasingly, some doctors are now happy to allow you to tape record your discussions to jog your memory of what he or she said. Research has shown that having such a recording is a great help to yourself, and your family, in following a doctor's observations or advice.

• Keep a diary of important events or issues between visits to
  the doctor, so that you can discuss these at your next visit.

**Not only when I was having diagnostic tests for MS,
but also when I had a subsequent attack, my neurologist
admitted me to hospital for a few days; yet my friend
who has MS – who has a different neurologist – has
hardly spent any time in hospital at all. Why is that?**

First it may well have been to do with undertaking tests or treatments particular to you, especially if you are already participating in a clinical trial (see Chapter 17). Secondly, in an acute
phase of the MS, especially with new symptoms, observing and
assessing how those symptoms develop can be valuable in terms
of planning your future care. Thirdly, neurologists may have
particular preferences about how they approach and manage
people with MS.

17
Research

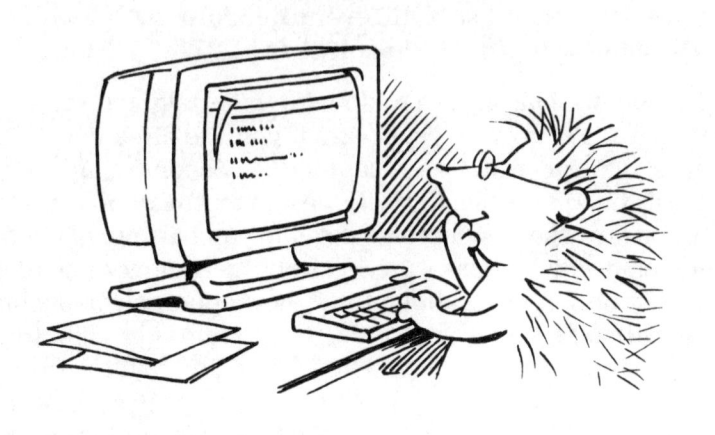

Research on the causes, possible cures and ways of managing MS has increased dramatically in recent years. Much of the information that has advanced our understanding of MS has come from what is called basic research – general knowledge of how the brain and central nervous system work and, more recently, how susceptibility to disease may be transmitted genetically.

Genetics

Scientists say that they have recently discovered the MS gene. What does that mean for me and for my MS?

Worldwide investigation into the human genome, i.e. the complete genetic blueprint of human life, has been vast; now variations in a number of areas of the genome have been linked with the presence of MS. However, this search is still very much in its early stages, and at the moment it seems that there may be several genes, and in more than one area of the genome, which individually and together raise the risk of developing MS, or increase susceptibility to it. We may have to wait several more years for clarification of the exact genetic influences on different types of MS, and several years beyond that for anything that might influence the onset or the course of the disease.

Will all this research into the genetics of MS mean that scientists will also find a cure for MS, like they have for cystic fibrosis?

Well, first we must be cautious about the 'cure' for cystic fibrosis (CF). The initial claims of a cure for CF appeared over 10 years ago, when a single defective gene for this disease was identified. These claims have not yet lived up to their promise, and the idea of 'gene therapy' is still being tested. So, although the discovery of the single gene for CF is the first major success story for molecular biology, the 'cure' is still under development. In the case of MS it seems most likely that the disease results from a combination of the action of several genes (unlike the single gene causing CF) and environmental factors.

What are the specific areas of research in MS at the moment?

There are broadly five kinds of scientific research being under-taken in relation to MS at present:

- The systematic study of the distribution and patterns of MS in different communities and countries – usually known as **epidemiological research** – involves asking questions about whether MS is more common in one geographical area than another, or is decreasing or increasing in a particular population over time, and what factors might explain these differences.

- Research which investigates the backgrounds of people with the disease: in the best studies using **'case-control' methods** (where each person with MS in the study is individually compared to another person without MS of a similar age and gender, and who has other factors in common with them), there has been no single disease, symptom or illness that has stood out universally as differentiating people with and without MS. Occasionally a modest link seems to have been found with, say, a childhood illness, but the link is usually at such a low level, and is then disputed by other researchers, that it is hard to say whether there is any 'real' association, much less a causative link. One of the problems of this kind of research is that it has to be done retrospectively, relying essentially on people's memories of their past illnesses, and this has proved a very unreliable source of information.

- **Laboratory-based research** focuses on questions related to the development of MS, for example why and how it affects specific nervous system tissue, where researchers often work at the level of individual cells; or what the possible genetic differences are between people with and without MS where blood or tissue types are examined.

- **Clinical research** on patients seeks to answer questions about what is often called the 'natural development' of MS in individuals, through the investigation of particular symptoms and signs that develop in those individuals over time, and what consequences these have for people's ability to function in everyday life. Related clinical research concentrates on questions about the effectiveness of potential therapies for MS, commonly undertaken through clinical trials – often after extensive safety testing in the laboratory.

- More studies are taking place in what is often called **applied research** in relation to MS. In the absence of a cure, much of this research is investigating how, for example, physiotherapy or speech therapy can reduce the impact of symptoms, or how far psychological support or counselling can help people to manage their symptoms better.

A lot of the time I keep hearing about the importance of 'clinical trials' in relation to MS. What is a clinical trial?

A clinical trial is a formal scientific means of testing the safety or the effectiveness of a drug or other treatment, either against another drug or treatment, or against what is called a *placebo*, i.e. an inactive substance which cannot be distinguished from the 'real' or active drug by people who are taking part in a trial nor by the doctors who are administering it. This way the drug can be tested for efficacy compared to the other drug or substance.

In a clinical trial of a potential therapy for MS, usually one group of patients (the experimental group) receives the active drug or the drug being tested, and another group (the control group) receives either the drug against which it is to be compared, or the placebo, the inactive substance. The two groups of patients should be as similar as possible at the outset of the trial, so that the drug alone will make the difference between the groups.

Various characteristics of the two groups of people will be measured before, during and after the trial – typically measures of disability, the number of MS 'attacks' or 'relapses' people have had, and other things such as blood cell counts or hormone levels. It is always hoped, of course, that the trial will show that the group which has received the active drug will do better.

I am keen to participate in clinical trials in order to get the chance of taking a new drug. How do I make sure I receive the new drug?

If you participate in a clinical trial for MS, note that you will not necessarily receive the new drug – but you will probably have **a 50–50 chance** to take it if you are randomized to the 'treatment group'.

However, there are several reasons why it is still worth your while joining a clinical trial, even if you are not given the new drug by being randomized to a comparison group:

• To be frank, it is likely that you will receive more careful clinical assessment and support, than you otherwise would do, if you participate in a clinical trial, whether you receive the new drug or not. This is because all those participating have to be meticulously and regularly monitored.

- You will almost certainly gain from the 'placebo effect' – the benefits which are often felt by people taking even an inactive substance – whatever you are taking in the trial.

- You would have the altruistic satisfaction of participating in a trial which would benefit others, even if you do not have the new drug yourself.

- Often trial procedures allow standard tried and tested therapies to continue if, for example, you have an attack or exacerbation during the trial.

- More frequently now, trials compare one drug with another, not just with a placebo substance. In these trials you would receive an active drug, whichever group you were in. Indeed the comparison drug will already have been shown to be effective in managing some aspects of MS, and often the new drug is one in which only a marginal additional assistance for MS is hoped for – but not yet known.

Will I have to pay for the drugs I receive in a trial?
No. You should not be asked to pay for any drugs you receive during the trial. There is an issue, however, that sometimes arises, and that is at the conclusion of a trial, when a new drug may be found to be effective, and participants wish to continue taking it. You might have to negotiate this through your usual doctor. In many cases this may be difficult because new drugs may be very expensive to obtain privately, and they may not yet be licensed for clinical use in the NHS outside a trial.

How do I get onto a list to participate in new drug trials?

Depending on the type of clinical trial concerned, people are used from many different sources, but the largest source of all are people with MS already under the care of neurologists, or those who are attending hospital clinics. In Britain the major means of recruitment is usually directly through your neurologist. When they are notified of a particular trial or are undertaking a trial themselves, they will investigate their own lists of people with MS to see whether any are suitable for the trial. You may then be contacted and asked if you would be prepared to participate. Of course, you can make your neurologist aware of your interest in clinical trials at one of your assessment meetings or by letter. Increasingly, in the United States, trials are more widely advertised through specialist centres and publications, and people can apply directly to participate, but in Britain this more open process of recruitment is still in its infancy.

Where can I find out more about current research in MS?

There are several sources. Which you use depends on your own inclinations, and indeed your own resources! The most important source of reliable and accurate scientific research on MS is that contained in scientific, and especially neurological, journals. Recent key issues and findings on MS from the journals can be obtained through computer searches, often through ordinary libraries, using one of the major medical databases such as 'Medline'. The MS Society provides information on research both past and present, and is increasingly putting out press statements and information in its regular newsletter on major current research issues.

If you have access to the World Wide Web, you can visit the Web sites of the MS Society in Britain and the United States; use one of the 'Search Engines' on the Web to trawl for updates on MS, and other sources of information; or join one of the growing number of Newsgroups in which people exchange information about new developments and other issues about MS. These latter groups are particularly important in terms of contact with other people with MS, and are often likely to be amongst the first sources of information about all kinds of developments, both scientific and non-scientific. Web addresses are currently changing too fast to permit any sensible listing here, but one source which is likely to be with us for some time is the Usenet News Group at news://alt.support.mult-sclerosis – this group hosts 50–100 messages per day and includes announcements about new Web pages and updates about existing pages.

You may also go to a good public library (a regional centre rather than a local library) and search for books on MS. Most libraries, including most local public libraries now have computer terminals for keyword and title searches. Library staff are often keen to help with difficult searches and to help locate specific information.

18

The Multiple Sclerosis Society

written by Jan Hatch,
Director of MS Services, MS Society

The Multiple Sclerosis (MS) Society has been mentioned several times in the answers to the questions in this book. It is the largest national organization in the UK providing support, information and services to anyone affected by multiple sclerosis.

This chapter will give you basic information about the Society and its work. If you would like further details of the services offered or how to get in touch with a local branch or support group, please contact the Society's national office at the address given in Appendix 1.

Background and aims

Sir Richard Cave founded the MS Society in 1953. His wife had MS and, following the example of an American woman called Sylvia Lawry, he decided to set up an organization in the UK with two main aims:

- to raise money to fund research into the cause of MS and to find the cure for MS;

- to provide support to people living with MS, including carers, families and friends as well as health and social care professionals.

These remain the aims of the MS Society today. The Society has over 45000 members, 370 branches, 19 regions and offices in Scotland and Northern Ireland. The help and support is offered to people affected by MS regardless of whether or not they are members. People with MS are actively encouraged to participate at every level in the organization. Many of the Society's Trustees have MS or care for someone with MS. People with MS are also very active as volunteers at the regional and branch level.

National offices

The national offices for England/Wales, Scotland and Northern Ireland offer a wide range of support for people affected by MS. This includes a freephone helpline, telephone counselling services, an information service, booklets and information materials, advocacy and financial assistance, a network of respite and holiday care facilities and services and education programmes for health and social care professionals.

In addition, the staff and volunteers work to ensure that politicians, statutory authorities, health and social care providers and the general public have a clear and accurate understanding of the needs of people affected by MS. Public awareness programmes, campaigning and lobbying and the promotion of standards of care and service are an important part of the work done by the Society. People with MS and their carers and families are directly involved in all of these activities.

Branches

Branches of the MS Society provide a wide range of support and information. Offering opportunities for mutual support, information about local facilities and services, financial assistance, transport and fundraising, each branch is run by volunteers, many of whom have a personal interest or experience of MS.

Branches are a focal point for people with an interest in MS in each local community. In many places they are very influential in promoting improvements in the health and social care provided to people with MS and their families and friends. Sometimes this is done through providing services themselves but more often it is through advocating on behalf of individuals and lobbying for change with health and social service providers.

Service provision

Membership

As a member of the Society, everyone receives a copy of MS Matters, the Society's bimonthly magazine and newsletter. This publication is an important source of up-to-date information on research, treatments and therapies, symptom management, employment, specialist equipment and disability aids, developments in social security benefits, changes in health and social care policy. In addition, every issue features individuals with MS, carers and family members highlighting their experience of living with MS.

Membership also gives people the opportunity to participate in national and regional elections, national and local campaigns, and in surveys and research projects sponsored by the Society.

Support and information

The Society provides a wide range of support for everyone affected by MS, including carers, family members, friends, colleagues, employers, health and social care professionals.

The National Telephone Helpline is a freephone line and is available from 9am to 9pm, Monday to Friday. Offering a listening ear to people with MS and their families and friends, this service is confidential and anonymous. Specialists in symptom management, social security benefits, employment and support for those recently diagnosed are available to provide a comprehensive service. In addition, trained volunteers with MS also work on the line.

The information service provides comprehensive information on all aspects of MS and research to health and social care professionals, students and the general public. A wide range of booklets, information sheets, videos and audiotapes is also available. A comprehensive collection of books, articles, journals, CD-Roms and internet search facilities is also available.

Information about the provision of wheelchairs, specially adapted vehicles, home adaptations, specialist computer and other equipment is available. Help in dealing with health and social services is also provided, as is help in finding sources of financial support.

Assistance in dealing with problems with employment or discrimination or with the issues related to the Disability Discrimination Act is available. Conferences specifically for people with MS and carers are held every year dealing with subjects such as symptom management, employment, relationships and other issues of importance.

Finally, the Society is the largest provider of specialist respite and holiday care specifically for people with MS in the UK. There are a total of seven units in England and Scotland, four respite nursing centres and three holiday care hotels. In addition, many branches have specially adapted holiday chalets, caravans or cottages. In Leicestershire an innovative home-based respite care service is available to people who live in the area.

Research

The Society is the largest provider of research funding specifically for MS in the UK. Having invested over £30 million in biomedical research over the past 46 years, the Society is the largest funder of this type of research in Europe. Funds are also now being provided for research into treatments, therapies, care services and other aspects of living with MS. The Society works closely with other MS charities both in the UK and internationally, and is committed to ensuring that all research takes account of the needs of people living with MS. This commitment focuses on involving them at every stage of the research process and is an important innovation in the Society's approach to research.

Fundraising and public awareness

Fundraising is vital to the work of the Society. Branches have always had an important role in raising the money that is needed to provide services and support at the local level and to fund research. In addition, their efforts to raise public awareness of MS have ensured that the Society has a very high profile in most local communities.

The work of the national office is also very important in educating and informing the public about multiple sclerosis and its effects on people with MS and their families. Over 51% of the UK population know someone with MS and their willingness to provide financial support for the work of the Society is great.

Glossary

ACTH (adrenocorticosteroid hormone) This hormone reduces inflammation. Clinical trials in the 1970s and later showed that it reduced the length of relapses or exacerbations in MS. More recently, a different family of steroids (glucocorticosteroids) has been found to have fewer side effects, as well as generally being more effective. So ACTH is used less in MS than previously, although some neurologists feel that ACTH still has significant value in treating MS relapses.

action tremor An involuntary trembling or shaking of a muscle or muscle group which is more noticeable during movement than when the muscle is at rest, for instance when reaching for an object or taking a step. Some degree of tremor is normal for all people, but a tremor that interferes with ordinary activity may be a symptom of neuromuscular disorder.

activities of daily living (or ADLs) A set of activities essential to independent living, such as washing, dressing and eating. Some particular sets of activities, as well as formalized procedures for measuring the performance of those activities, have become established as assessments of the degree of disability caused by MS. Such ADL scores may be used to record the progress of MS, to assess domestic needs or to test the effects of drugs in clinical trials.

ambulant Able to walk unassisted, with or without a walking aid (a stick or frame, for instance).

anticholinergic drugs Such drugs are used in the management of urinary problems due to neurological impairment. The name refers to the way in which the drugs work by affecting the parasympathetic nervous system, reducing spasms (contractions) in the bladder and thus reducing the likelihood of involuntary or too frequent urination.

artefact effect   A coincidental association wrongly stated between two factors, but often explained by a third factor.

atrophy   Wasting away or reduction in tissue, particularly muscle tissue, following prolonged disuse.

auditory evoked response   An electrical signal in the brain that occurs in response to sound. Tests can reveal changes in the speed, shape and distribution of these signals which are indicative of a diagnosis of MS.

autoimmune disease   A disorder of the immune system in which the processes that usually defend against disease run amok and attack the body's own tissues (such as myelin, in the case of MS). Other autoimmune conditions include rheumatoid arthritis and lupus erythematosus. The systematic study of autoimmune diseases as a group is becoming an important part of research into MS.

benign MS   MS which is either mild (possibly displaying no active symptoms) or in which there is little or no evidence of progressively more severe symptoms.

beta-blockers   A class of drugs (known more fully as beta-adrenergic blocking agents) commonly used to treat high blood pressure, irregular heart beat and angina.

bipolar disorder   Known previously as manic-depressive disorder, a condition that is characterized by extreme and unpredictable mood swings.

blood–brain barrier (BBB)   The barrier separating the brain from the blood supplying it. In normal circumstances, essential nutrients can cross the barrier from the blood into the brain and waste products cross from the brain into the blood, but the cells of the brain are shielded from potentially harmful substances in the blood itself.

Borrelia burgdorferii   The Latin name for the infectious organism that causes Lyme disease, an entirely treatable infection spread by ticks, which has many symptoms in common with MS and can be mistaken for it.

bowel incontinence   *see* **faecal incontinence**

bowel regimen A programme involving changes in diet and timing of bowel movements designed to control faecal incontinence. Dietary changes include an increase in fibre and fluid intake to increase the bulk and to soften bowel movements, and a reduction in intestinal irritants such as coffee and alcohol. A bowel regimen may also employ laxatives and drugs to help complete emptying of the bowel at predictable times.

Candida albicans Also known as thrush, this is a fungus that is often present in the genitals, mouth and other moist parts of the body. Symptoms of candidiasis include irritation, itching, abnormal discharges and discomfort on passing water. Candidiasis can be effectively treated with antifungal drugs.

cardiovascular Relating to the heart and blood vessels.

cerebrospinal fluid (CSF) The fluid surrounding the spinal column and nerves supplying stimuli to the brain. The CSF contains proteins and tissue fragments that can aid the diagnosis of neurological disorders and differentiate MS from other conditions with similar or overlapping symptoms. A sample of CSF can be taken with a spinal tap (see **lumbar puncture**).

chi (qi) In Chinese medicine, the essential life-force or energy flowing in the body, imbalance of which results in the symptoms of disease or illness.

chronic progressive (or primary progressive) MS A type of MS characterized by a pattern of unremittingly and progressively more severe or widespread symptoms over time.

cognitive abilities Abilities to perform tasks related to thought processes – for instance problem-solving, recognition, memory and recall. Changes in cognitive ability are often subtle and not apparent without sophisticated testing. Cognitive tests may reveal evidence of changes due to MS.

cognitive issues A set of issues relating to such things as memory, information processing, planning and problem solving, which are of recent but rapidly growing significance to the study of MS.

computerized axial tomography (CAT or CT) scan A form of detailed X-ray imaging involving multiple exposures at different positions and angles throughout the same part of the body. Computerized manipulation of the exposures results in clear images of fine structures such as sclerotic plaques within the brain or spinal column.

contractures Shortening or shrinkage of tissue (such as connective or muscular tissue) which may result from inflammation caused by MS and which can restrict movement of joints. Exercises to maintain the flexibility of joints are particular important because contractures may be made worse by lack of joint use.

demyelination The biochemical process of damage to the protective sheath surrounding nerves, damage or loss of which leads to symptoms of MS. The breakdown of *myelin* leads to poor or weak messages to various parts of the body and may lead, in the case of MS, to the formation of plaques or scarring with hardened (sclerotic) tissue.

diplopia Double vision, resulting (in the case of MS) from impaired control of eye muscles.

electroencephalographic (EEG) recordings The measurement of the small electric charges generated by nerve signals within the brain, using electrodes placed harmlessly on the skin of the scalp.

epidemiology The study of patterns of birth, death and disease within and between human populations. Often epidemiological studies try to find relationships between the frequency of MS and variations in other factors (such as diet or exposure to infections).

essential fatty acids Important substances crucial to nervous system development and health mainly in the families of linoleic, linolenic and arachidonic acids. They cannot be synthesized by the body and must be obtained from the diet.

euphoria A strong sense of happiness or well-being, usually in response to a pleasurable stimulus. However, euphoria without such an obvious stimulus may occur in MS.

faecal (bowel) incontinence The involuntary release of faeces from the bowel, resulting from constipation and partial obstruction of the bowel or from diminished control of the anal sphincter. Treatment of faecal incontinence with a bowel regimen is often completely successful in preventing involuntary bowel movements.

familial component of disease A situation in which more relatives have the same disease than would be expected by chance. This can be

due to an inherited susceptibility to the disease (nature) or to the
environmental and other exposures that families inevitably share
(nurture).

family pedigrees   A family tree which details the number of instances of
disease amongst all members related to each other by blood. Pedigrees
are important in determining the mechanisms of genetic inheritance.

foot drop   A disorder in which, instead of the normal 'heel then toe'
pattern of walking, the toe touches the ground first, leading often to
tripping and falling. The condition results from weakness in the ankle and
foot muscles, caused by weakening of nervous system control of these
muscles.

frequency   The desire or need to empty the bladder often.

functional abilities   Ability to perform tasks. A number of objective
tests have been developed to assess the extent to which these abilities
may be affected by the progression of MS.

gait analysis   The study of exactly how people walk, which can be used
to assess the effects of MS. It can then be used to assess the effectiveness
of therapies, such as physiotherapy, in helping people to walk more
comfortably.

glucocorticosteroids   A family of drugs (including prednisone,
prednisolone, methylprednisolone) which, whilst produced naturally by
the adrenal gland, can be made synthetically. They have immunosuppressive and anti-inflammatory properties. They are replacing **ACTH**
for use in MS exacerbations.

hesitancy   An involuntary delay or inability to start urinating.

immunosuppressive drugs   Drugs which suppress the body's natural
immune responses. They have been widely used in MS because immune
responses are considered to be directed against the person's own body in
the disease.

improved case ascertainment   Sometimes people may have MS but it
has not been diagnosed. Improved case ascertainment is the increased
ability of the medical services to identify correctly such existing cases
which have been previously undetected.

incidence of disease   The measure of how often new cases of a disease are diagnosed within a population over a given time period. Incidence is usually reported per 100 000 people per year.

incontinence Loss of control of bladder or bowel function. Incontinence may result in occasional accidents or in more serious loss of voluntary control of urination or bowel movements.

inoculations *see* **vaccinations**

intramuscularly Injections within or into a muscle as opposed to intravenous (directly into a vein) injections.

labile Volatile or unstable. What is called 'emotional lability', i.e. unpredictable or changeable moods, occurs in some people with MS.

latitude effect An often-repeated observation in MS research that there is a relationship between the incidence of MS and the distance from the equator (or latitude in geography). In other words, the further you go from the equator, the more MS cases there are. The nature of the relationship has not been fully unravelled, and there are many explanations as to why it does exist.

licensed drugs Medicinal compounds licensed by the Committee on the Safety of Medicines for general use within medical practice in respect of particular illnesses – in other words, licensed drugs also have licensed purposes. Not all legally available drugs are licensed, such as new and untested drugs as well as some private treatments, supplements and complementary treatments.

lumbar puncture (spinal tap) A procedure in which a hollow needle is inserted into the spinal canal between two vertebrae in the lower back, in order to withdraw a sample of **cerebrospinal fluid** for biochemical analysis.

magnetic resonance imaging (MRI) A procedure in which a magnetic field, generated inside a large cylinder in which the person to be examined lies, produces detailed images of fine structures within the body. Unlike X-ray imaging, MRI can image soft tissue such as the brain, spinal column and blood vessels.

major depressive episode A state in which deep sadness and unhappiness may be accompanied by disturbances or major problems in appetite and sleep patterns, plus feelings of hopelessness, worthlessness and suicidal thoughts.

medical history   Literally, the file of notes and records about a patient and his or her medical events. The taking of a medical history (the interview in which a doctor asks how an illness or symptoms started) is a crucial first phase in the diagnosis of any condition. In the case of MS, where diagnosis can be a long, tedious and complex procedure, the collection of an accurate and complete medical history is of particular importance.

meridians   Lines of energy running through the body, connecting the different anatomical sites, upon which much traditional Chinese medicine is based.

motor symptoms   Symptoms relating to muscular movement and the control of motion. Motor symptoms are those symptoms of MS which result from various components of degeneration of nervous system function resulting from MS plaques.

multiple scleroses   Scleroses (or sclerotic plaques) are deposits of hardened tissue which can result from inflammation around nerves in many parts of the body. Some scleroses are temporary, and all people have scleroses which come and go. In MS, a sclerosis can result in abnormal and more permanent damage in many parts of the nervous system. In severe MS, there may be many of these scleroses causing loss of control of muscle function.

myelin   An electrical insulator covering nerve fibres which ensures that nerve messages are effectively transmitted to various parts of the body. *See also* **demyelination**

neurological examination   An evaluation of the function of the nervous system involving, often, a great number of individual examinations and tests. A neurological assessment is essential to the diagnosis of MS, which will (at least initially) involve the elimination of other, often more serious or immediate, conditions with similar symptoms. These may include the taking of a relevant **medical history**, **auditory** and **visual evoked response** tests as well as examination of reflexes, senses and functional abilities. **MRI** and **CAT** scans may be employed where it is thought their results would significantly aid the diagnosis. An examination of **cognitive function** (such as memory and problem solving) is becoming more uncommon. A full neurological assessment may take place on several occasions and be spread over many weeks or months.

neuron A nerve cell.

NICE (National Institute of Clinical Excellence) This independent body has recently been established by the British Government to assess the effectiveness of healthcare interventions in relation to their cost. The intention is that only interventions (including drugs) approved by NICE will be available through the NHS.

nocturia The desire or need to pass urine during the night, often disturbing restful sleep.

nystagmus An involuntary, jerking movement of the eyes resulting (in the case of MS) from damage to the nervous system. Nystagmus can result in severe visual problems that make reading extremely tiring or difficult.

oligoclonal banding The banding is distributed in the spinal fluid of a large proportion (90%) of people with MS, although it is not limited to just those people. The banding indicates abnormal levels of antibodies.

optic neuritis Inflammation of the optic nerve behind the eye. Optic neuritis can result in temporary loss of vision, as well as pain and tenderness.

paresis Weakness or partial paralysis of muscles.

population ageing A term for the general trend, in all industrialized nations, towards greater life expectancy. Increased life expectancy leads inevitably to a greater proportion of people at all older ages, a greater dependency ratio (the ratio of employed people to children and retired people), and a greater proportion of the population with long-term medical needs. Population ageing and the resulting increased demand for health services will become an increasingly important political issue over coming decades.

prevalence A measure of the proportion of the population with a given condition, often expressed as so many cases of the condition for each thousand people of the population. This measure allows comparison of the frequency of the condition between populations of different sizes.

primary progressive MS *see* **chronic progressive MS**

prognosis An educated assessment of the likely future course of a medical condition and its effects. No prognosis can ever be more than a good guess based on prior experience, and may include both best and worst case outcomes.

progressive neurological disease   A disease of the nervous system that becomes progressively more severe or has more widespread symptoms over time.

qi   *see* **chi**

recall bias   The tendency of those people, when answering questions about past events, to selectively remember past events and circumstances. For instance, people who have a disease affecting their ability to walk may selectively remember more illnesses or accidents affecting their legs compared to other people who may have had an equal number of illnesses or accidents. Recall bias can be a significant problem when researchers are trying to discover past events which may have caused a disease.

relapsing-remitting MS   A type of MS which is characterized by relapses, i.e. a relatively rapid increase in symptoms, followed by remissions in which there is a partial or full recovery from these untreated symptoms. In some cases complete recovery may occur from all symptoms, but in most cases recovery is partial. Relapses may recur every few months or may be as much as years apart.

scotoma A 'gap' or disturbance in one part of your visual field.

secondary progressive MS   A type of MS in which, following initially benign or relapsing-remitting MS, symptoms then begin to progress steadily.

selective recall   *see* **recall bias**

sensory symptoms   Symptoms which involve a problem with one of the senses – touch, taste, smell, hearing and sight. All senses may be affected in MS, although visual and auditory disturbances are most frequently reported and are most likely to impact on activities of daily living.

sequelae   The indirect effects of a condition. For instance, urinary tract infections and bed sores are not caused by MS, but can result from immobility and being bedbound, and are more common amongst people with severe symptoms of MS.

shiatzu A form of massage based on the pressure treatment (acupressure) of points associated with acupuncture treatment.

spasticity Stiffness or tension in muscles that is not caused by excessive exercise, and in MS is usually caused by the continuing effect of poor nervous system control of the relevant muscles.

spinal tap *see* **lumbar puncture**

subcutaneously Under the skin, e.g. a subcutaneous injection is given in the tissues immediately beneath the skin.

tremor An involuntary shaking or trembling of muscles, at rest or (more commonly in MS) during movement.

trigeminal neuralgia This is acute pain associated with disorder of the trigeminal nerve – the nerve supplying the cheek, lips, gums and chin. The pain is usually intense, stabbing, brief and associated with only one side of the face.

urgency The desire or need to pass urine immediately. Urgency is not necessarily associated with a full bladder, but is nevertheless almost impossible to ignore.

Uthoff's phenomenon A temporary disturbance of vision that may follow vigorous exercise.

vertigo A disorientating sensation of unsteadiness. The world often appears to be spinning. It may sometimes be described as a dizzy spell. Vertigo results from a disturbance of the fluid in the inner ear or from a disorder of the nerve carrying signals from the inner ear to the brain. Even a simple but unfamiliar situation (such as sailing) can cause vertigo in a healthy person, leading to nausea or vomiting.

vestibular system The system of balance that operates through fluid-filled canals in the inner ear and the nerve carrying signals from the inner ear to the brain.

visually evoked response An electrical signal in the brain that occurs in response to sight of an image. EEG recordings of responses to test patterns, often of regular patterns of black and white squares or lines of different sizes, can be used to determine the nature and location of certain abnormalities of brain function.

voiding Literally, emptying. Voiding is usually applied to bowel motions and passing urine. Incomplete voiding refers to the situation where, after a motion or urination, the bowel or bladder is not emptied completely.

Appendix 1

Useful addresses

National and regional MS societies

The Multiple Sclerosis Society of Great Britain & Northern Ireland
   Headquarters
25 Effie Road
Fulham
London SW6 1EE
Tel: (020) 7610 7171
Fax: (020) 7736 9861 or (020) 7610 9912
Freephone Helpline: 0808 800 8000 (open from Mon–Fri 9am–9pm)
www.mssociety.org.uk
See Chapter 18.

The Multiple Sclerosis Society in Scotland
2a North Charlotte Street
Edinburgh EH2 4HR
Tel: (0131) 225 3600
Fax: (0131) 220 5188

The Multiple Sclerosis Society Northern Ireland Office
34 Annadale Avenue
Belfast BT7 3JJ
Tel: (028) 9064 4914

The Multiple Sclerosis Society Telephone Counselling Lines
(24-hour service via referral from answerphones listed below)
London: (020) 7222 3123
Midlands: (0121) 476 4229
Scotland: (0131) 226 6573

International MS societies

Multiple Sclerosis Society of Canada
250 Bloor Street East
Suite 1000
Toronto
Ontario M4W 3P9
Canada

The Multiple Sclerosis Society of Ireland
Royal Hospital
Donnybrook
Bloomfield Avenue
Morehampton Road
Dublin 4
Ireland
Tel: (00 353) 1 269 4599
Fax: (00 353) 1 269 3746
The MS Society of Ireland offers a caring and informative service,
which includes a telephone advice and counselling line. It provides a
countrywide network of local branches and counsellors, and funds
specialized community workers. Publications include an information
pack on all aspects of MS. It is also a member of the International
Federation of MS Societies (IFMSS).

International Federation of Multiple Sclerosis Societies (IFMSS)
10 Heddon Street
London W1R 7LJ
Tel: (020) 7734 9120
Fax: (020) 7287 2587
www.ifmss.org.uk
IFMSS coordinates the research and welfare projects of its 34 national
MS Society members. It also organizes an annual world conference and
publishes *Update*, a quarterly magazine, and *MS Management* twice a
year.

Other MS-related organizations

British Trust for the Myelin Project
Douglas Cottage
2 Eshiels
Peebles EH45 8NA
Tel: (01721) 720546
Fax: (01721) 723474
The British branch belongs to an international network that is focused
on accelerating research into the repair of myelin and reduction of
disabilities. The Myelin Project is committed to sharing the scope and
results of the research it funds.

Jooly's Joint
www.mswebpals.org
A free Website for people with MS.

MS Healing Trust
Tel: (0121) 744 7167
The MS Healing Trust exists to maximize the healing potential in
people with MS. It runs a weekly clinic at Shirley, attended by doctors
and complementary therapists, and an information service.

MS Nerve Centre
Tel: (0117) 928 2463
The MS Nerve Centre runs a national helpline and information service
about resources as well as funding research.

Multiple Sclerosis Research Trust
Spirella Building
Bridge Road
Letchworth SG6 4ET
Tel: (01462) 476700
Fax: (01462) 476710
This trust provides positive information about MS, especially for those who are newly diagnosed, and for professionals working to meet the needs of those with MS.

Multiple Sclerosis Resource Centre
7 Pear Tree Business Centre
Pear Tree Rd
Stanway
Colchester CO3 5JN
Tel: (01206) 505 4444
Freephone: (0800) 783 0518
The MS Resource Centre offers advice on all aspects of living with MS day to day. Its magazine *Pathways* and an information pack are available on request.

Naomi Branson Research Trust
Barclays Venture Centre,
The Science park, University of Warwick
Coventry CV4 7EZ
Tel: (024) 7641 3671
As well as researching into other neurological disorders, the Naomi Branson Research Centre makes available diagnostic testing for MS.

Multiple Sclerosis Therapy Centres

Many excellent MS therapy centres operate throughout Great Britain and Northern Ireland offering information, advice and practical help. Such centres provide a wide range of therapies regarded as useful in managing MS. These include physiotherapy, yoga, speech therapy, chiropody, diet control, continence advice, reflexology, aromatherapy and counselling. Some centres operate their own hyperbaric oxygen treatment chambers.

Association of Therapy Centres
(Scotland)
Tayside Friends of Arms
Unit 12b
Peddie St
Dundee DD1 5LB
Tel/Fax: (01382) 566283

Federation of MS Therapy
Centres
Bradbury House
155 Barkers Lane
Bedford MK41 9RX
Tel: (01234) 325781
Fax: (01234) 365242
www.mstherapycentres.
demon.co.uk

Northern Association of MS
Therapy Centres
The Village
Forth Avenue
Trafford Park
Manchester M17 19B
Tel: (0161) 872 3422
Fax: (0161) 876 4593

Other useful addresses

AbilityNet (formerly
Computability Centre)
PO Box 94
Warwick CV34 5WS
Tel: (01026) 312847
Fax: (01926) 407425
Freephone Advice Line:
0800 269545
www.abilitynet.co.uk

AbilityNet (formerly Foundation
for Communication for the
Disabled)
Beacon House
Pryford Roas
West Byfleet KT14 6LD
Tel: (01932) 336512
Fax: (01932) 336513
www.abilitynetfreeserve.co.uk
Supplies computer systems designed for disabled people.

Age Concern England
Astral House
1268 London Road
London SW16 4ER
Tel: (020) 8679 8000
Fax: (020) 8765 7211
www.ace.org.uk

Age Concern Scotland
113 Rose Street
Edinburgh EH2 3DT
Tel: (0131) 220 3345

Alliance for Cannabis
 Therapeutics
P.O. Box CR14
Leeds LS7 4XF
Fax: (0113) 237 1000

AREMCO Swivel Cushions
Grove House
Lenham ME17 2PX
Tel: (01622) 858502
Fax: (01622) 850532

Association of Community Health
 Councils for England and Wales
Earlsmead House
30 Drayton Park
London N5 1PB
Tel: (020) 7609 8405
Fax: (020) 7700 1152
www.achcew.org.uk

Association of Crossroads Care
 Attendant Schemes
10 Regent Place
Rugby CV21 2PN
Tel: (01788) 573653

Association of Disabled
 Professionals
170 Benton Hill
Wakefield Road
Horbury WF4 5HW
Tel/Fax: (01924) 283253
www.adp.org.uk

Association of Professional
 Music Therapists
36 Pierce Lane
Fulbourn
Cambs CB1 5DL
Tel: (01223) 880377

Association of Reflexology
27 Old Gloucester Street
London WC1N 3XX
Tel: (0990) 673320
Fax: (01989) 567676
www.reflexology.org/aor

B-Active
see address for Outset
Provides training help for people
with disabilities in Bedfordshire,
under Government New Deal
scheme.

Benefits Agency
Chief Executive's Office
Room 4C06
Quarry House
Quarry Hill
Leeds LS2 7UA
Tel: (0113) 232 4000

British Acupuncture Council
63 Jeddo Road
London W12 9HQ
Tel: (020) 8735 0400
Fax: (020) 8735 0404
www.acupuncture.org.uk

British Association for
   Counselling
1 Regent Place
Rugby CV21 2PJ
Tel: (01788) 550899
Fax: (01788) 562189
Information line: (01788) 578328
www.counsellingco.uk

British Complementary Medicine
   Association
Kensington House
33 Imperial Square
Cheltenham GLS0 1QZ
Tel: (0116) 282 5511
Fax: (01242) 227765

British Council for Disabled
   People
Litchurch Plaza
Litchurch Lane
Derby DE24 8AA
Tel: (01332) 295551
Fax: (01332) 295580
www.bcodp.org.uk
Information: (01332) 298288
Minicom: (01332) 295581
Support for organizations of
disabled people

British Herbal Medicine
   Association (BHMA)
Sun House
Church St
Stroud GL5 1JL
Tel: (01453) 751389

British Holistic Medical
   Association
Tel: (01273) 725951

British Homeopathic Association
   (BHA)
27A Devonshire St
London W1N 1RJ
Tel: (020) 7935 2163
www.nhsconfed.net/bha

British Medical Acupuncture
   (BMAS)
Newton House
Newton Lane
Whitley
Warrington WA4 4JA
Tel: (01925) 730727
Fax: (01925) 730492
www.medical-acupuncture.co.uk

British Reflexology Association
   (BRA)
Monks Orchard
Whitbourne WR6 5RB
Tel: (01886) 821207
Fax: (01529) 822017
www.britreflex.co.uk

British Society for Disabilty
and Oral Health
Dr Janice Fiske
Floor 26 Guy's Dental School
London SE1 9RT
Tel: (020) 7955 5000 ext. 3295
Fax: (020) 7955 2676

British Sports Association
for the Disabled
Mary Glen Haig Suite
Solecast House
13–27 Brunswick Place
London N1 6DX
(020) 7490 4919

British Wheel of Yoga
1 Hamilton Place
Boston Road
Sleaford NG34 7ES
Tel: (01529) 306851
www.members.aol.com/wheelyoga

Canon UK Ltd
Canon House
Manor Road
Wallington
Surrey
SM6 0AJ
Tel: (020) 8773 3173
Fax: (020) 8773 6095
www.canon.co.uk

Carers National Association
20/25 Glasshouse Yard
London EC1A 4JT
Tel: (020) 7490 8818
Fax: (020) 7490 8824
www.carersuk.demon.co.uk

Chester-Care
Sidings Road
Low Moor Estate
Kirkby-in-Ashfield
Notts NG17 7JZ
Tel: (01623) 757955
Fax: (01623) 755585

Chivers Large Print Books
Chivers Press Ltd
Windsor Bridge Road
Bath BA2 3AX
Tel: (01225) 335336
Fax: (01225) 310771

Citizen Advocacy Information
and Training (CAIT)
164 Lea Valley Technopark
Ashley Road
Tottenham Hale
London N17 9LN
Tel: (020) 8880 4545

Citizens Advice Bureaux
(National Association –
NACAB)
Myddelton House
115–123 Pentonville Road
London N1 9LZ
Tel: (020) 7833 2181
Fax: (020) 7833 4371
www.nacab.org.uk
Will provide details of your local
Citizens Advice Bureau.

Citizens Advice Scotland
26 George Square
Edinburgh EH8 9LD
Tel: (0131) 667 0156

Community Health Councils
see Association of
Community Health Councils

Community Service Volunteers
237 Pentonville Road
London N1 9NJ
Tel: (020) 7278 6601

Compassionate Friends
53 North Street
Bedminster
Bristol BS3 1SN
Helpline: (0117) 953 9639
Support for bereaved parents
and siblings

Computability Centre
see AbilityNet

Continence Campaign
c/o LSA
110 St Martins Lane
London WC2 N4DY
Tel: (020) 7841 5451
Fax: (020) 7841 5424

Continence Foundation
2 Doughty Street
London EC1N 2PH
Helpline (020) 7831 9831
(Mon-Fri 9am–4.30pm)

Council for Disabled Children
8 Wakely Street
London EC1V 7QE
Tel: (020) 7843 6058
Fax: (020) 7278 9512
(National Children's Bureaux):
www.ncb.org.uk

Counsel and Care
Lower Ground Floor
Twyman Hosue
16 Bonny Street
London NW1 9PG
Tel: (020) 7485 1566
(10.30am–4.00pm)
Advice line (local rate):
(0845) 300 7585
Fax: (020) 7267 6877

Crossroads Caring for Carers
10 Regent Street
Rugby CV21 2PN
Tel: (01788) 573653
Fax: (01788) 565498
Professional support to carers
and people with care needs;
services in England, Wales and
N. Ireland.

Crossroads Scotland Care
Attendant Scheme
24 George Square
Glasgow G2 1EG
Tel: (0141) 226 3793
Fax: (0141) 221 7130

Cruse Bereavement Care
126 Sheen Raod
London TW9 1UB
Tel: (020) 8940 4818
Bereavement Line:
(020) 8352 7227
Counselling, support groups,
practical information and advice.

DIAL UK
Park Lodge
St Catherine's Hospital
Tickhill Road
Balby
Doncaster DN4 8QN
Tel: (01302) 310123
Fax: (01302) 310404
www.members.aol.com./dialuk

Disabilities Trust
First Floor
Market Place
Burgess Hill RH11 9NP
Tel: (01444) 239123
Fax: (01444) 244978
www.disabilitys-trust.org.uk
Care and accommodation for
physically disabled people.

Disability Alliance
First Floor East
Universal House
88–94 Wentworh Street
London E1 7SA
Tel: (020) 7247 8776
Fax: (020) 7247 8765
Offers a rights service.
Disability Discrimination Act
Information Line: (0345) 622633

Disability Discrimination Act
Representation and Advice
Project (DDARAP)
11 Broadway House
Jackman Street
London E8 4QY
Tel: (020) 7254 8434

Disability Equipment Register
4 Chatterton Road
Yate
Bristol BS37 4BJ
Tel: (01454) 318818
Fax: (01454) 883870
www.disareg.dial.pipex.com
Nationwide service to buy and
sell used disabled equipment.

Disability Law Service
2nd Floor, High Holborn House
52–54 High Holborn
London W31V 6RL
Tel: (020) 7831 8031/7740
Provides legal advice.

Disability Now
12 Park Crescent
London W1N 4EQ
Tel: (020) 7636 5020

Disability Scotland
Princes House
5 Shandwick Place
Edinburgh EH2 4RG

Disability Sport England
13–27 Brunswick Place
London N1 6DX
Tel: (020) 7490 4919
Fax: (020) 7490 4914

Disabled Access to Technology
   Association
Broomfield House
Bolling Road
Bradford BD4 7BG
Tel: (01274) 370019

Disabled Christians' Fellowship
213 Wick Road
Brislington
Bristol BS4 4HP
Tel: (0117) 983 0388
Fellowship by correspondence,
cassettes, local branches,
holidays, youth section, local
workshop and day centre.

Disabled Drivers' Assocation
National Headquarters
Ashwelthorpe
Norwich NR16 1EX
Tel: (01508) 489449
Fax: (01508) 488173
www.disabled-drivers.org.uk
Self-help association aiming for
independence through mobility.

Disabled Drivers Insurance
   Bureau
10 Greencoat Place
London SW3P 1PR
Tel: (020) 7306 0606

Disabled Drivers' Motor Club
Cottingham Way
Thrapston
Northamptonshire NN14 4PL
Tel: (01832) 734724
Fax: (01832) 733816
web.uk.online.co.uk.ddmc
Offers advice on all problems for
the disabled motorist and family.

Disabled Drivers' Motorists Club
Tel: (01743) 761889

Disabled Living Centres Council
1st Floor Winchester House
11 Cranmer Road
London SW9 5E
Voice and Text: (020) 7820 0567
Coordinates work of Disabled
Living Centres UK wide. List of
centres available.

Disabled Living Foundation
380/384 Harrow Road
London W9 2HU
Tel: (020) 7289 6111
Fax: (020) 7266 2922

Disabled Motorists Federation
National Mobility Centre
Unit 2a
Atcham Estate
Shrewsbury SY4 4UG
Tel: (01743) 761181

Disablement Income Group (DIG)
5 Archway Business Centre
19–23 Wedmore Street
London N19 4RZ
Tel: (020) 7263 3981
Promotes the financial welfare of
disabled people.

DVLA
Drivers Medical Unit
Longview Road
Morriston
Swansea SA99 1TU
Tel: (01792) 783686

Equal Opportunities Commission
Overseas House
Quay Street
Manchester M3 3HN
Tel: (0161) 833 9244
Fax: (0161) 835 1657
www.eocorg.uk

Family Fund Trust
PO Box 50
York YO1 2ZX
Tel: (01904) 621115

Family Service Units
207 Old Marylebone Road
London NW1 5QP
Tel: (020) 7402 5175

Family Welfare Association
501–505 Kingsland Road
London E8 4A
Tel: (020) 7254 6251
Fax: (020) 7249 5443

Foundation for Communication
for the Disabled *see* AbilityNet

Gardening for the Disabled Trust
c/o F Seton
The Freight
Cranbrook N17 3PG
Tel: (01580) 712196

GEMMA
BM Box 5700
London WC1N 3XX
National Friendship network of
disabled and non-disabled lesbian
and bisexual women.

General Osteopathic Council
Osteopathy House
176 Tower Bridge Road
London SE1 3LU
Tel: (020) 7357 6655

Gingerbread (Organization for
lone parent families)
16–17 Clerkenwell Close
London EC1R OAA
Tel: (020) 7336 8183
Advice: (020) 7336 8184

Handihols
see Special Family's Trust

Help for Health Trust
Highcroft
Romsey Road
Winchester SO22 5DH

Health Development Agency
(for visits 9.00–5.00)
Trevelyan House
30 Great Peter Street
London SW1P 2HW
Tel: (020) 7222 5300
Fax: (020) 7413 0339 (for
   catalogue)

Holiday Care Service
2nd Floor
Imperial Buildings
Victoria Road
Horley RH6 7PZ
Tel: (01293) 774535
Holiday information and support.

Holiday Homes Trust (Scouts)
Baden Powell House
Queen's Gate
London SW7 5JS
Tel: (020) 7584 7030
Fax: (020) 7590 5103
Source of low cost, self-catering
holidays for disabled and
disadvantaged people (no
scouting connection necessary).

Holidays (Help the
   Handicapped– 3H Fund)
147a Camden Road
Tunbridge Wells TN1 2RA
Tel: (01892) 547474
Fax: (01892) 524703

Home Care Support
382 Hillcross Avenue
Mordon SM4 4EX
Tel: (020) 8542 0348

Horticultural Therapy
   see THRIVE

Huntleigh Health
310–312 Dallow Rd
Luton LU1 1TD
Tel: (01582) 413104
Fax: (01582) 459100

Incapacity Action
65 Casimir Road
Clapton
London E5 9NU
Campaigning group working for
rights for long-term sick and
disabled people.

Independent Living Alternatives
Trafalgar House
Grenville Place
London NW7 3SA
Tel: (020) 8906 9255

Independent Living Fund
PO Box 183
Nottingham NG8 3RD
Tel: (0115) 942 8191
Fax: (0115) 929 3156

Institute for Complementary
   Medicine
PO Box 194
London SE16 1QZ
Tel: (020) 7237 5165
Fax: (020) 7237 5175
www.icmedicine.co.uk

John Grooms Association for
Disabled People
50 Scrutton Street
London EC2A 4PH
Tel: (020) 7452 2000
Fax: (020) 7452 2001
www.johngrooms.org.uk
A charity providing a range of
residential care, housing, holidays
and work across the UK.

Keep Able Ltd
For a mail order catalogue,
write to:
FREEPOST
Wellingborough
Northants NN8 6BR

Shops at:
11–17 Kingstown Road
Staines TW18 4QX
and
Sterling Park
Pedmore Road
Brierley Hill DY5 1TA
and
Fleming Close
Park Farm
Wellingborough NN8 6UF

Law Centres Federation
Duchess House
18–19 Warren Street
London W1P 5DB
Tel: (020) 7387 8570
Fax: (020) 7387 8368
www.lawcentres.org.uk

Also
3rd Floor Arundel Court
177 Arundel Street
Sheffield S1 2NU
Tel: (0114) 278 7088
Information on your nearest
Law Centre.

Law Society
114 Chancery Lane
London WC2A 1PL
Tel: (020) 7320 5793
Fax: (020) 7316 5697
Group for solicitors with
disabilities.

Leonard Cheshire Foundation
30 Millbank
London SW1P 2QW
Tel: (020) 7828 1822

Liberty (The National Council
for Civil Liberties)
21 Tabard Street
London SE1 4LA
Tel: (020) 7403 3888

Listening Books
12 Lant Street
London SE1 1QH
Tel: (020) 7407 9417
Fax: (020) 7403 1377
www.listening-books.org.uk
Provides listening books on tape
for adults and children.

Long-Term Medical Conditions
Alliance (LMCA)
c/o Unit 212
16 Baldwins Gardens
London EC1N 7RJ
Tel: (020) 7813 3637
Fax: (020) 7813 3640
www.lmca.co.uk
Aims to improve the quality of life
of people with long-term medical
conditions.

Low Pay Unit
27–29 Amwell Street
London EC1R 1UN
Employment Rights Helpline:
(020) 7713 7583

Mediair Marketing Services
72 High Street
Poole BH15 1DA
Tel: (01202) 671545

Medical Alert Foundation
1 Bridge Wharf
156 Caledonian Road
London N1 9UU
Tel: (020) 7833 3034
Fax: (020) 7713 5653

Mobility Assessment Centres
Details about your nearest centre
can be obtained from:
Mobility Advice and Information
Service (MAVIS)
'O' Wing Macadam Avenue
Old Wokingham Road
Crowthorne RG11 6AU
Tel: (01344) 661000
Fax: (01344) 661066
www.mobilityunit.detr.gov.uk/
mavis.htm
or
Disabled Drivers' Motor Club
(*see above*)

Mobility for Disabled People
(Joint Committee)
c/o Muscular Dystrophy Group
7–11 Prescott Place
London SW4 6BS
Liaising and campaigning body on
mobility, access and transport.

Mobility Information Service,
National Mobility Centre
Unit 2a Atcham Estate
Shrewsbury SY4 4UG
Tel: (01743) 761889
Information on mobility. Driving
assessment for disabled drivers.

Motability
Goodman House
Station Approach
Harlow
Essex CM20 2ET
Tel: (01279) 635666
Fax: (01279) 632000

National Centre for Independent
    Living
250 Kennington Lane
London SE11 5RD
Tel: (020) 7587 1663
Provides information,
consultancy and training on
personal assistance and direct
payments.

National Childbirth Trust
Alexandra House
Oldham Terrace
London W3 6NH
Tel: (020) 8992 8637

National Disabled Person's
    Housing Service (DPHS)
Brunswick House
Deighton Close
Wetherby LS22 7GZ
Tel: (01904) 653888
Promoting and supporting the
creation of local disabled person's
housing services.

National Gardens Scheme
Hatchlands Park
East Clandon
Guildford GU4 7RT
Tel: (01483) 211535
Fax: (01483) 211537
www.ngs.org.uk

National Institute of Medical
    Herbalists
56 Longbrook Street
Exeter EX4 6AH
Tel: (01392) 426022
Fax: (01392) 498963
www.btinternet.com./~nimh/

NCH Action for Children
85 Highbury Park
London N5 1UD
Tel: (020) 7226 2033
Fax: (020) 7226 2537
www.nchafc.org.uk
Community and residential
projects for children with
disabilities.

Opportunities for People with
    Disabilities
1 Bank Buildings
Princes Street
London EC2R 8EU
Tel/Fax: (020) 7726 4961
www.opportunities.org.uk

Open University
Regional Disability Coordinator
Walton Hall
Milton Keynes MK7 6AA
Tel: (01908) 652255
Fax: (01908) 659044
www.open.ac.uk

Outset
6th Floor Cresta House
Alma St
Luton LU1 2PL
Tel: (0870) 2000 001
Centre for training courses for
people with disabilities and long-
term illness/unemployment.

Partially Sighted Society
PO Box 322
Doncaster DN1 2XA
Tel: (01302) 323132
London office: (020) 7372 1551

Patients' Association
PO Box 935
Harrow HA1 3YJ
Tel: (020) 8423 9111
Fax: (020) 8423 9119
Helpline (020) 8423 8999
www.patients-association.com
Help and advice for patients.
Leaflets and self-help directory
available.

Pensions Advisory Service
    (OPAS)
11 Belgrave Road
London SW1V 1RB
Tel: (020) 7233 8080
Fax: (020) 7233 8016
www.opas.org.uk
Free help to people with pension
problems.

PHAB England
Summit House
Wandle Road
Croydon CR0 1DF
Tel: (020) 8667 9443
Fax: (020) 8681 1399
Clubs and holidays to bring
disabled and able-bodied people
together.

Queen Elizabeth's Foundation
    for Disabled People
Leatherhead Court
Leatherhead
Surrey KT22 0BN
Tel: (01372) 842204
Fax: (01372) 844072
www.qufd.org
Provides vocational and social
rehabilitation and training,
information services and driving
assessments.

RADAR (Royal Association for
    Disability and Rehabilitation)
12 City Forum
250 City Road
London EC1V 8AF
Tel: (020) 7250 3222
Fax: (020) 7250 0212
www.radar.org.uk
Minicom: (020) 7250 4119

Rail Unit for Disabled Passengers
    Switchboard
Tel: (020) 7928 5151

Red Cross Society
9 Grosvenor Crescent
London SW1X 7EJ
Fax: (020) 7235 6315

RELATE (National Marriage
    Guidance)
Herbert Gray College
Little Church Street
Rugby CV21 3AP
Tel: (01788) 573241
Fax: (01788) 535007
www.relate.org.uk

Remploy Ltd
415 Edgeware Road
London NW2 6LR
Tel: (020) 8235 0500
Fax: (020) 8235 0501

Research Council for
    Complementary Medicine
505 Riverbank House
1 Putney Bridge Approach
London SW6 3JD
Tel: (020) 7384 1772
Fax: (020) 7384 1736
www.rccm.org.uk

Riding for the Disabled
    Association
Lavinia Norfolk House
Avenue 'R' NAC
Stoneleigh park
Warwickshire CV8 2LY
Tel: (0247) 669 6510
Fax: (0247) 669 6532
Provides the opportunity of riding
and driving to disabled people.

Rights Now Campaign
c/o RADAR (*see above*)
Pressure group for civil rights for
disabled people.

Royal London Homeopathic
    Hospital
Great Ormond Street
London WC1N 3HR
Tel: (020) 7837 8833

Sequal Trust
3 Ploughmans Corner
Wharf Road
Ellesmere SY12 0EJ
Tel/Fax: (01691) 624222
Assessment and provision of
communication skills

Shaftesbury Society
16 Kingston Road
London SW19 1JZ
Tel: (020) 8239 5555
Fax: (020) 8239 5580
www.shaftesburysoc.org.uk
Residential centres, schools,
colleges and holiday centres for
disabled people.

Shirley Price Aromatherapy Ltd
Essentia House
Upper Bond Street
Hinkley
Leicestershire LE10 1RS
Tel: (01455) 615466
Fax: (01455) 615054
www.shirleyprice.aroma.co.uk

SKILL
National Bureau for Students
  with Disabilities
Chapter House
18–20 Crucifix Lane
London SE1
Tel: (0800) 328 5050
Fax: (020) 7450 0650
www.skill.org.uk

Snowden Award Scheme
22 City Business Centre
Horsham RH13 5BA
Tel: (01403) 211252
Fax: (01403) 271553
Bursaries to help physically
disabled students with the
additional costs of further
education or training.

Special Collection
J D Williams
Freepost
PO Box 123
Manchester M99 1BN
Tel: (0161) 237 1200
Fax: (0161) 238 2626
A mail order catalogue of fashion
clothing selected for people with
dressing difficulties.

Special Family's Trust (formerly
  Handihols)
Erme House
Station Rd
Plympton
Plymouth PL7 3AU
House exchange or hospitality
scheme for disabled people.

SPOD (Association to Aid
  the Sexual and Personal
  Relationships of People
  with a Disability)
286 Camden Road
London N7 0BJ
Tel: (020) 7607 8851/2
Fax: (020) 7700 0236

SSAFA Forces Help
Special Needs Advisor
19 Queen Elizabeth Street
London SE1 2LP
Tel: (020) 7403 8783 or 7962 9698
Fax: (020) 7403 8815

Stress Management Training
  Institute
Foxhills, 30 Victoria Ave
Shanklin
Isle of Wight PO37 6LS
Tel: (01983) 868166
Fax: (01983) 866666
www.smti.org

Taking a Break *see* King's Fund

Talking Newspapers Association
  UK
National Recording Centre
Heathfield TN21 8DB
Tel: (01435) 866102
Fax: (01435) 865422
www.tnauk.org.uk

Telecottage Association
Freephone: (0800) 616008
Support network for people who
work from home.

THRIVE
Horticultural Therapy
Sir Geoffery Udall Centre
Beech Hill
Reading RG7 2AT
Tel: (0118) 988 5688
Fax: (0118) 988 5677
www.thrive.org.uk
Advice service to disabled
gardeners.

Tripscope
The Courtyard
Evelyn Road
London W4 5JL
Tel: (020) 8994 9294
Fax: (020) 8994 3618

Ulverscroft Large Print Books
F A Thorpe Publishing Ltd
The Green, Bradgate Road
Anstey LE7 7FU
Tel: (0116) 236 4325

Winged Fellowship Trust
Angel House
30/32 Pentonville Road
London N1 9XD
Tel: (020) 7833 2594
Fax: (020) 7278 0370
www.wft.org.uk

JJ Wright, National Organizer
Hazeldene
Ightham
Sevenoaks TN15 9AD
Tel: (01732) 883818
Makes or adapts aids, when not
commercially available, for
disabled people at no charge to
the disabled person.

Yoga for Health Foundation
Ickwell Bury
Biggleswade SG18 9EF
Tel: (01767) 627271
Fax: (01767) 627266

Appendix 2

Useful publications

Publications from the MS Society

MS Matters, the Society's newsletter is published six times a year (and also available on tape cassette), free to members. They also publish many useful booklets and pamphlets such as:

Complementary therapies
Coping and continent
Employing people with multiple sclerosis
Guide to staying in work (for employee)
Has your Mum or Dad got MS?
Making the most of life with MS
MS and healthy eating
MS and social security benefits
MS and your home
People with MS in long-term care
Sources of support
Standards of healthcare for people with MS
Treating MS symptoms
Understanding MS research
What is MS?

Other publications

See Appendix 1 for addresses of organizations mentioned here, and the list at the end of this book of other useful publications by Class Publishing. Class Publishing will be publishing further books on MS – please contact them for more information at the address given on p.iv.

Accessible holidays in the British Isles – a guide for disabled people. Updated annually

Age Concern. *Legal arrangements for managing financial affairs.* Factsheet Number 22

Barret, Michael. *Sexuality and multiple sclerosis*, published by MS Society of Canada

Benz, Cynthia. *Coping with multiple sclerosis*, published by Vermilion, 1996

Berriedale-Johnson, M & Davies, A. *Cook it yourself: cooking with a physical disability* published by Cedar

BT guide for disabled people (Available free from any BT shop by dialling Freefone (0800) 800150 [voice] or (0800) 243123 [text]. The guide can also be supplied in large print, braille or audiocassette tape.)

Burnfield A. *Multiple sclerosis – a personal exploration*, published by Souvenir Press, 1996

Carers National Association
Caring for someone at home
Getting help to adapt your home
Getting the most from your primary care team
How do I get help?
How to get my carer's assessment
Juggling your job and caring
Residential and nursing home care
Taking a break
Young carers power pack

Charities digest, published by the Family Welfare Association (updated every year)

Cornell, Susie. *Complete MS body manual*, available from PO Box 1270, Chelmsford, CM2 6BQ, 1996

Counsel and Care. *What to look for in a private or voluntary registered home* (Fact sheet No 5)

Darnbrough, Ann & Kinrade, Derek. *Directory for disabled people*, published by Wendy Botwright, Prentice Hall, Campus 400, Maylands Avenue, Hemel Hempstead HP2 7EZ, Tel: (01442) 882058

Department of Health. *Choosing a care home*, published by DoH (available from your local Health Authority)

Department of Health. *Health and advice for the traveller*, published by DoH (available from Post Offices)

Department of Transport. *Door to door*, available free of charge from the Mobility Advice and Vehicle Information Service (MAVIS)

Employment: guidance and code of practice. Stationery Office, London

Fildes, Susan. *Eating and MS – information and recipes*, published by MS Resource Centre, 1994

Fitzgerald, Geraldine & Briscoe, Fenella. *Recipes for health for MS*, published by Thorsons, 1996

Graham, Judy. *MS, pregnancy and parenthood*, published by MS Resource Centre, 1996

Guide to grants for individuals in need, published by Directory of Social Change (updated every other year)

Halper, June & Holland, Nancy. *Comprehensive nursing care in multiple sclerosis*, published by Demos Vermande, 1997

Health Education Board Scotland. *Coping with dementia. Handbook for carers*, published by Woodburn House, Canaan Lane, Edinburgh EH10 4SG

Historic houses, castles and gardens, published by Johansens, London (updated regularly)

Holiday care guide to accessible travel, published by the Holiday Care Service

Karr, KL. *Taking time for ME: How caregivers can deal effectively with stress*, published by Prometheus Books

Koher, Nancy. *Caring at home*, published by National Extension College, 18 Brooklands Avenue, Cambridge CB2 2HN

Llewellyn, R & Davies, A. *Grow it yourself: gardening with a physical disability*, published by Cedar

Loder, Cari. *Standing in the sunshine*, published by Century, 1996

Mackie, Carole & Brattle, Sue. *Me and my shadow*, published by Aurum Press, 1999

Mandelstam, Michael. *How to get equipment for disability*, published by Jessica Kingsley Publishers, 116 Pentonville Road, London N1 9JB, Tel: (020) 7833 2307

Matthews, WB (editor). *McAlpine's multiple sclerosis*, published by Churchill Livingstone, 1991 (2nd edition)

The National Gardens Scheme handbook (updated annually)

National Trust handbook (for members; updated annually)

Patterson, Judith. *Disability rights handbook*, published by Disability Alliance Educational and Research Association, London

RADAR factsheets
Copies of the following factsheets are available from RADAR.
Telephone for latest prices:

1. *Motoring with a wheelchair*
2. *Exemption from vehicle excise duty (VED)*
3. *Relief from VAT and car tax*
4. *Driving licences*
5. *Assessment centres and driving instruction*
6. *Insurance*
7. *Motoring accessories*
8. *Cash help for mobility needs*
9. *Discounts and concessions available to disabled people on the purchase of cars and other related items*
10. *Car control manufacturers, suppliers and fitters*

RICA. *Equipment for an easier life*, published by RICA

Segal, Julia. *Emotional reactions to MS*, published by the MS Resource Centre, 1994

Sibley W.A. (ed.) for the National MS Society of America. *Therapeutic claims in multiple sclerosis*, 5th edition, published by Demos Vermande Publishers, 1999

Thomas, Richard. *Multiple sclerosis – the natural way*, published by Element, 1995

Wates, Michael. *However will you cope?* (Discusses experiences of disabled mothers), published by National Childbirth Trust, 1996

With a little help, published by the Disabled Living Foundation

Yarrow, Michael. *Places that care*, published by Mediair Marketing Services

Index

Have you found **Multiple sclerosis at your fingertips** practical and useful? If so, you may be interested in other books from Class Publishing.

Allergies at your fingertips
Dr Joanne Clough £14.99
At last – sensible practical advice on allergies from an experienced medical expert.
> *'An excellent book which deserves to be on the bookshop of every family.'* – Dr Csaba Rusznak, Medical and Scientific Director, British Allergy Foundation

Asthma at your fingertips £14.99
Dr Mark Levy, Professor Sean Hilton and Greta Barnes MBE
This book shows you how to keep your asthma – or your family's asthma – under control, making it easier to live a full, happy and healthy life.
> *'This book gives you the knowledge. Don't limit yourself.'* – Adrian Moorhouse MBE, Olympic Gold Medallist

Alzheimer's at your fingertips £14.99
Harry Cayton, Dr Nori Graham, Dr James Warner
At last – a book that tells you everything you need to know about Alzheimer's and other dementias.
> *'An invaluable contribution to understanding all forms of dementia'.* – Dr Jonathan Miller CBE, President, Alzheimer's Disease Society

Cancer information at your fingertips £14.99
Val Speechley and Maxine Rosenfield
Recommended by the Cancer Research Campaign, this book provides straight-forward and positive answers to all your questions about cancer.

Diabetes at your fingertips £14.99
Professor Peter Sonksen, Dr Charles Fox and Sister Sue Judd
461 questions on diabetes are answered clearly and accurately – the ideal reference book for everyone with diabetes.
> *'I have no hesitation in commending this book'* – Sir Harry Secombe CBE, President of the British Diabetic Association

Heart health at your fingertips
NEW! £14.99
Dr Graham Jackson
This practical handbook, written by a leading cardiologist, answers all your questions about heart conditions.
> *'Contains the answers the doctor wishes he had given if only he'd had the time.'* – Dr Thomas Stuttaford, *The Times*

High blood pressure at your fingertips
NEW SECOND EDITION! £14.99
Dr Julian Tudor Hart with Dr Tom Fahey
The authors use all their years of experience as blood pressure experts to answer your questions on high blood pressure.
> *'Readable and comprehensive information'* – Dr Sylvia McLaughlan, Director General, The Stroke Association

Parkinson's at your fingertips
NEW SECOND EDITION! £14.99
Dr Marie Oxtoby and Professor Adrian Williams
Full of practical help and advice for people with Parkinson's disease and their families. This book gives you the information and the confidence to tackle the challenges that PD presents.
> *'An unqualified success'* – Dr Andrew Lees, Consultant Neurologist, The National Hospital for Neurology and Neurosurgery

Stop that heart attack!
NEW! £14.99
Dr Derrick Cutting
The easy, drug-free and medically accurate way to cut your risk of having a heart attack dramatically. Even if you already have heart disease, you can halt and even reverse its progress by following Dr Cutting's simple steps. Don't be a victim – take action NOW!

PRIORITY ORDER FORM

Cut out or photocopy this form and send it (post free in the UK) to:

Class Publishing Priority Service   **Tel: 01752 202301**
FREEPOST (PAM 6219)   **Fax: 01752 202333**
Plymouth PL6 7ZZ

Please send me urgently   *Post included*
(tick boxes below)   *price per copy (UK only)*

☐ **Multiple sclerosis at your fingertips** (ISBN 1 872362 94 X)	£17.99
☐ **High blood pressure at your fingertips** (ISBN 1 872362 81 8)	£17.99
☐ **Diabetes at your fingertips** (ISBN 1 872362 79 6)	£17.99
☐ **Heart health at your fingertips** (ISBN 1 872362 79 X)	£17.99
☐ **Parkinson's at your fingertips** (ISBN 1 872362 96 6)	£17.99
☐ **Stop that heart attack!** (ISBN 1 872362 85 0)	£17.99
☐ **Allergies at your fingertips** (ISBN 1 872362 52 4)	£17.99
☐ **Asthma at your fingertips** (ISBN 1 872362 67 2)	£17.99
☐ **Cancer information at your fingertips** (ISBN 1 872362 56 7)	£17.99
☐ **Alzheimer's at your fingertips** (ISBN 1 872362 71 0)	£17.99

TOTAL   _____

Easy ways to pay

Cheque: I enclose a cheque payable to Class Publishing for £ _____

Credit card: Please debit my ☐ Access   ☐ Visa   ☐ Amex   ☐ Switch

Number _____ Expiry date _____

Name _____

My address for delivery is _____

_____

Town _____ County _____ Postcode _____

Telephone number (in case of query) _____

Credit card billing address if different from above _____

_____

Town _____ County _____ Postcode _____

Class Publishing's guarantee: remember that if, for any reason, you are not satisfied with these books, we will refund all your money, without any questions asked. Prices and VAT rates may be altered for reasons beyond our control.